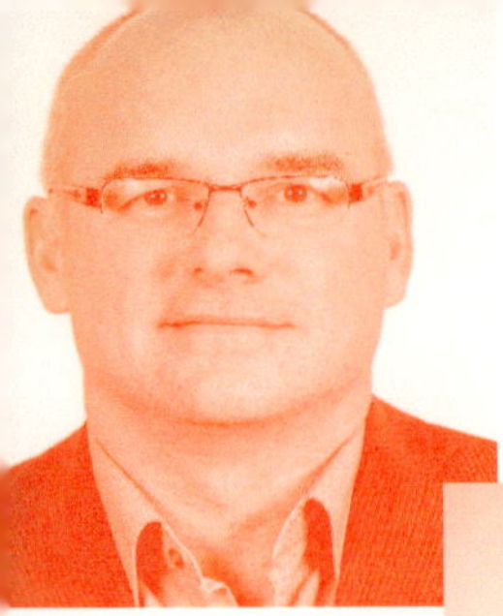
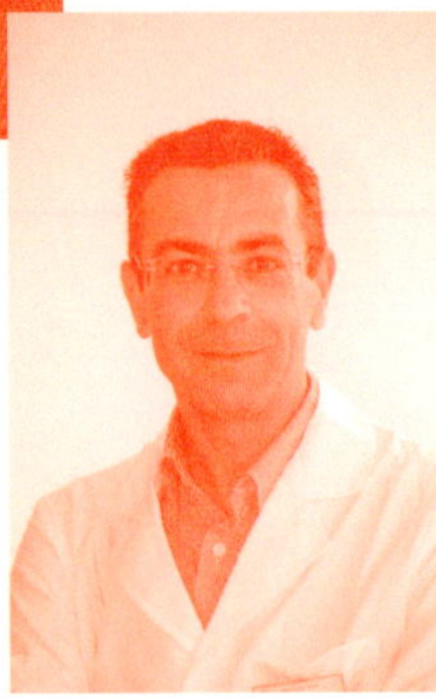
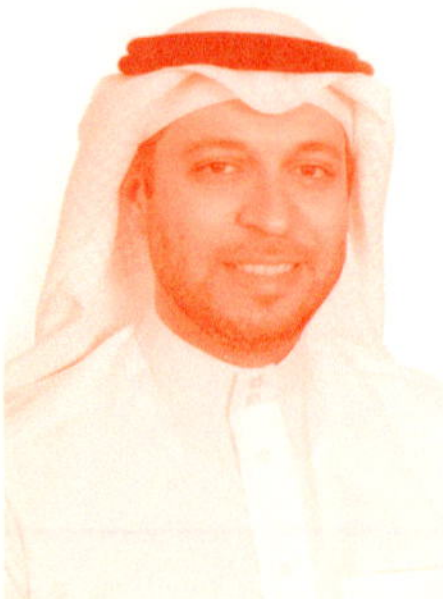
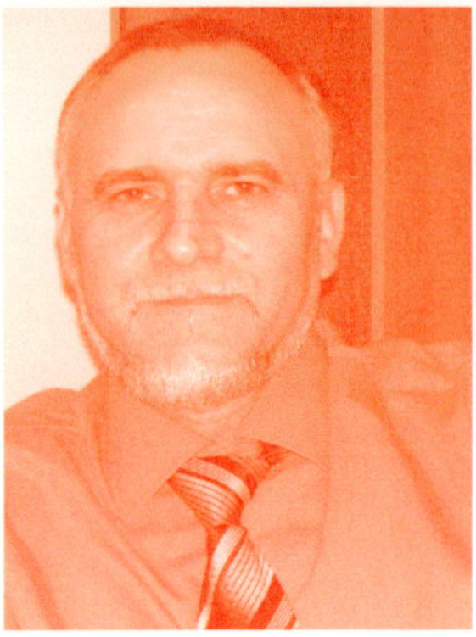
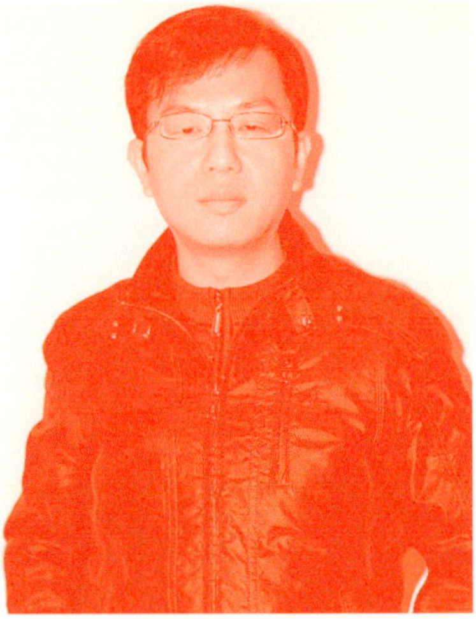
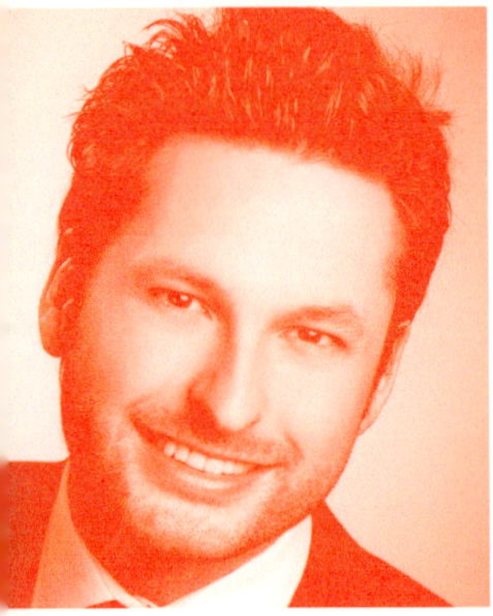
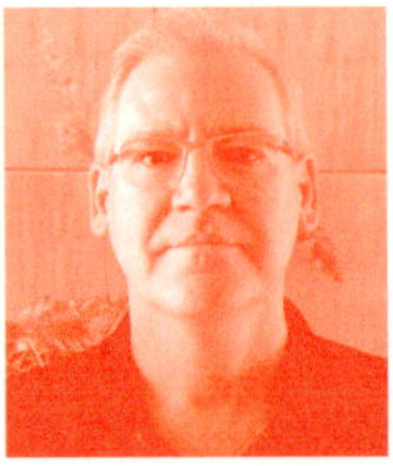

IntechOpen

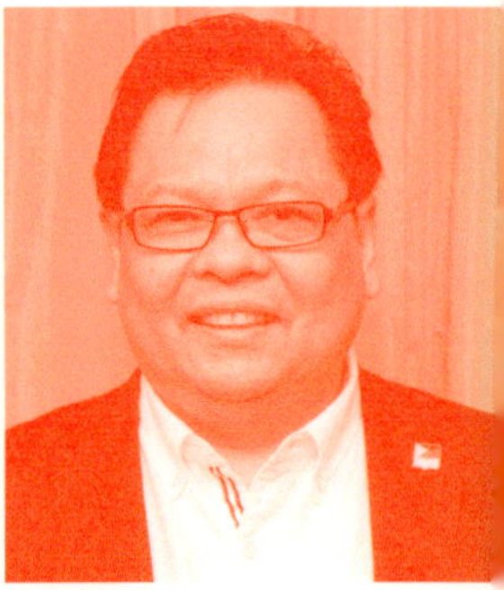
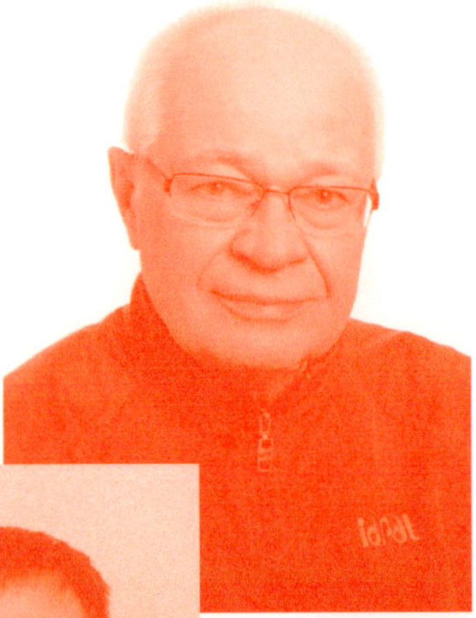
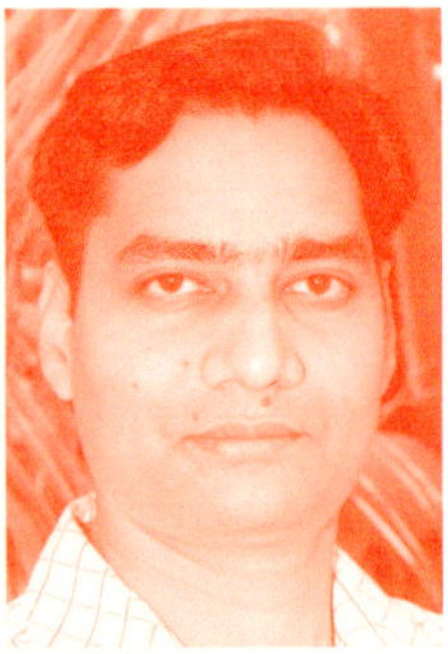
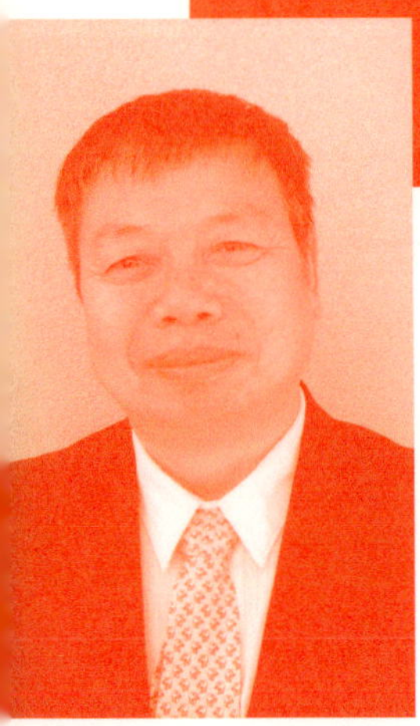
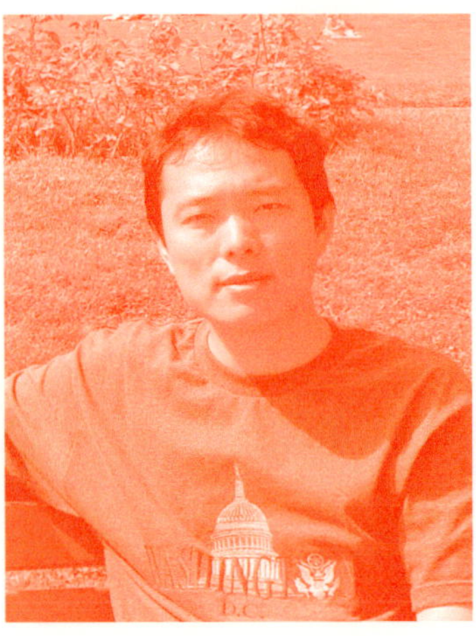
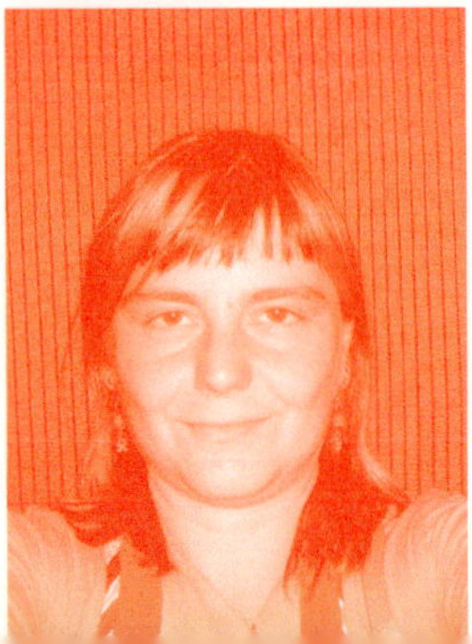

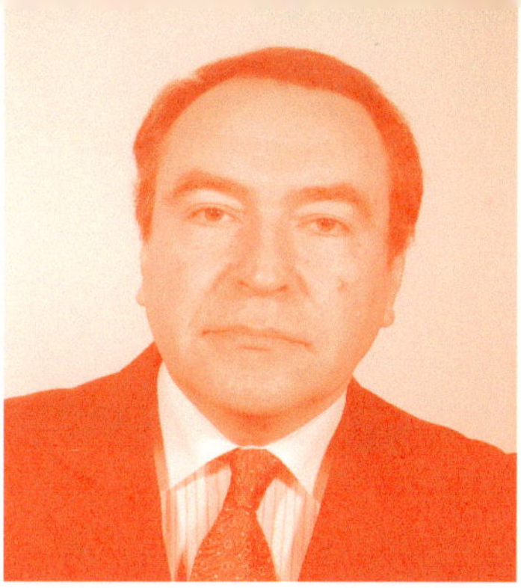
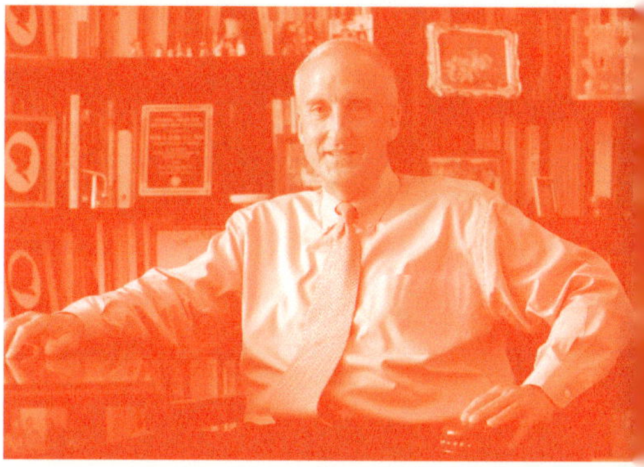
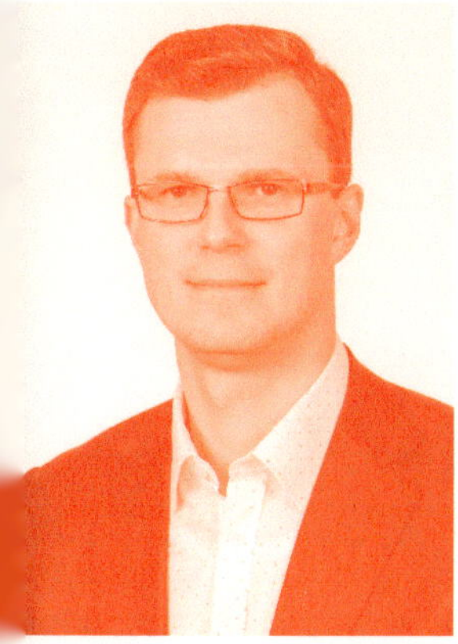
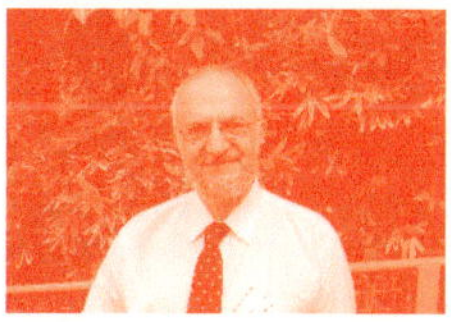
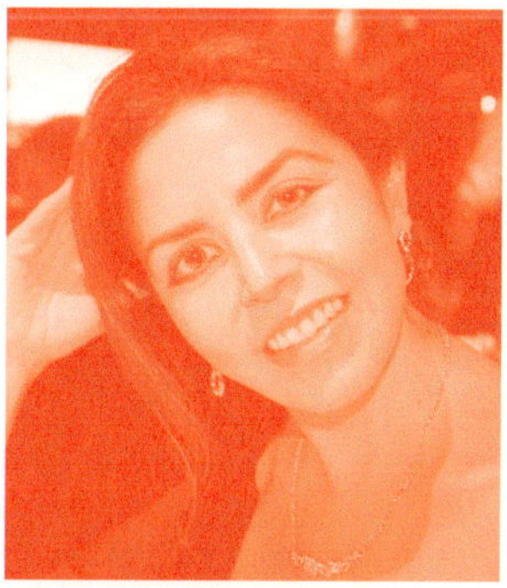

Supporting open minds since 2005

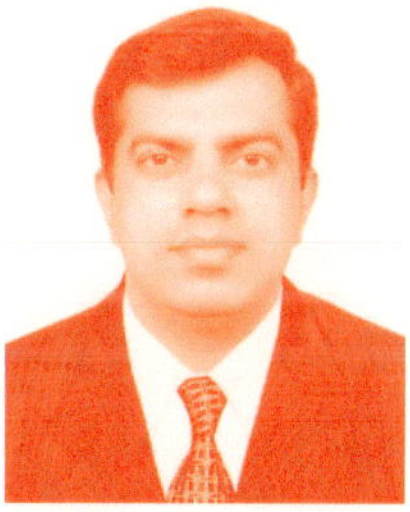
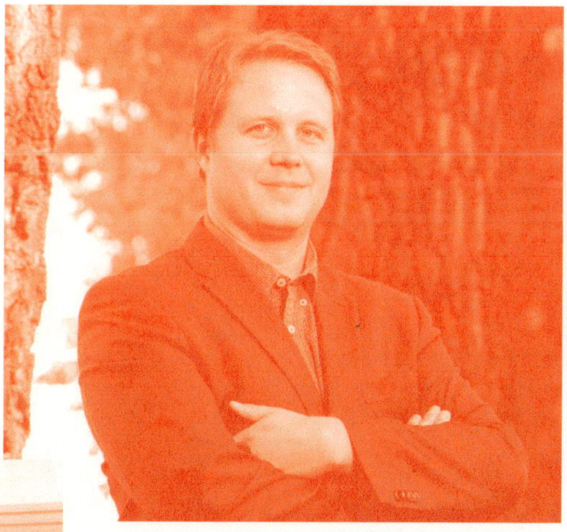
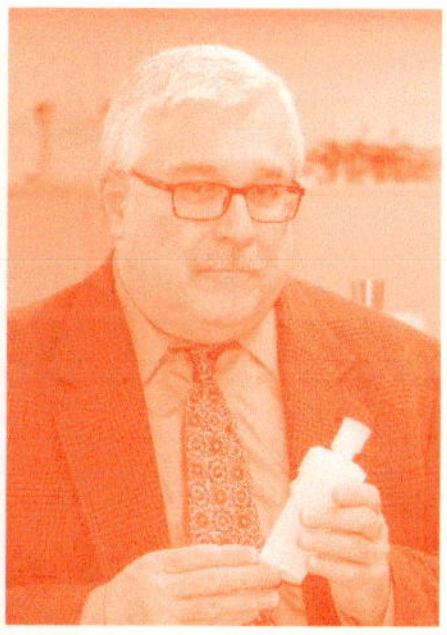
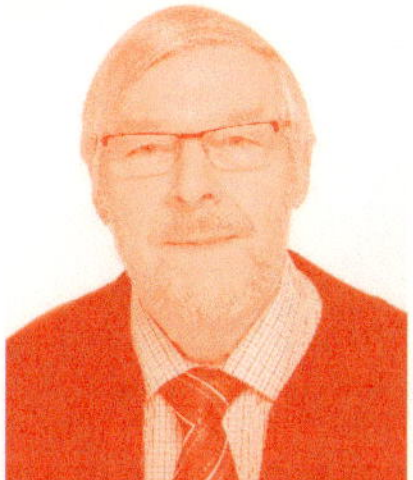
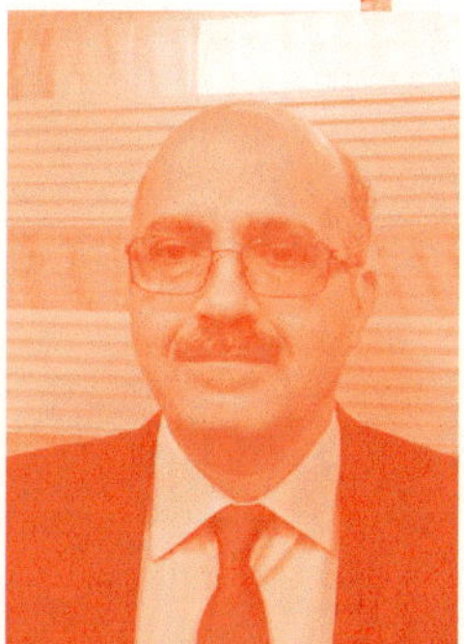
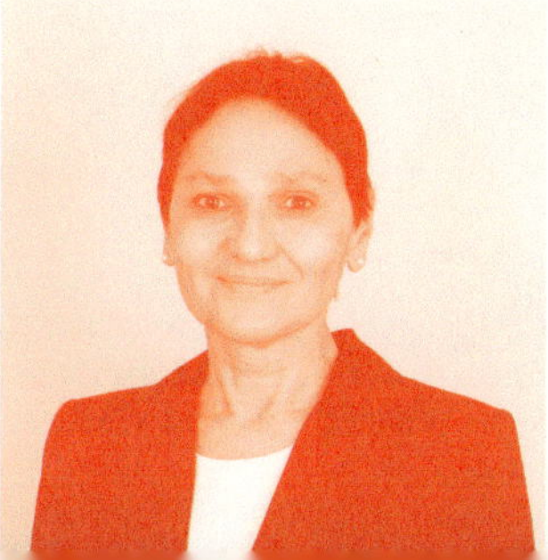
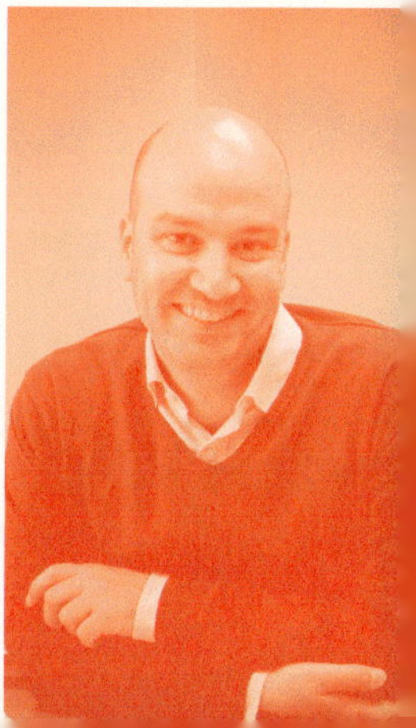

Adipose Tissue - An Update
http://dx.doi.org/10.5772/intechopen.80248
Edited by Leszek Szablewski

Part of IntechOpen Book Series: Physiology, Volume 4
Book Series Editor: Angel Catala

Contributors
Alina Kurylowicz, Rajan Singh, Shehla Pervin, Miguel L Batista Jr., Felipe Henriques, Alexander H. Bedard, Sara Al-Ghadban, Bruce Bunnell, Karen Herbst, Mohamed Elrayess, Haya Al-Sulaiti, Alex Domling, Dhara Patel, Palash Mandal, Leszek Szablewski

First published in London, United Kingdom, 2019 by IntechOpen
IntechOpen is the global imprint of INTECHOPEN LIMITED, registered in England and Wales, registration number: 11086078, 7th floor, 10 Lower Thames Street, London, EC3R 6AF, United Kingdom
Printed in Croatia

British Library Cataloguing-in-Publication Data
A catalogue record for this book is available from the British Library

Additional hard and PDF copies can be obtained from orders@intechopen.com

Adipose Tissue - An Update
Edited by Leszek Szablewski
p. cm.
Print ISBN 978-1-83880-121-2
Online ISBN 978-1-83880-122-9
eBook (PDF) ISBN 978-1-83962-541-1
ISSN 2631-8261

For EU product safety concerns:
IN TECH d.o.o., Prolaz Marije Krucifikse Kozulić 3, 51000 Rijeka, Croatia, info@intechopen.com or visit our website at intechopen.com.

IntechOpen Book Series
Physiology
Volume 4

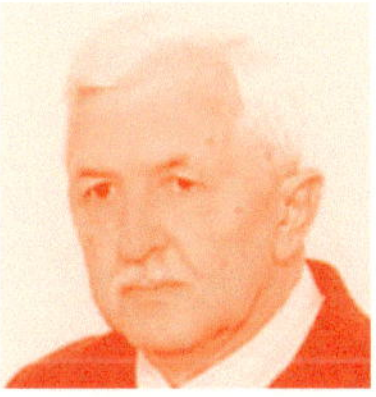

Leszek Szablewski is a professor of medical sciences. He received his MS in the Faculty of Biology from the University of Warsaw and his PhD degree from the Institute of Experimental Biology, Polish Academy of Sciences. He habilitated in the Medical University of Warsaw, and obtained his degree of professor from the President of Poland. Professor Szablewski is the Head of Chair of the Department of General Biology and Parasitology, Medical University of Warsaw. He has published over 80 peer-reviewed papers in journals such as *Journal of Alzheimer's Disease*, *Biochimica Biophysica Acta Reviews on Cancer*, *Biological Chemistry*, *Journal of Biomedical Science*, *Diabetes/Metabolism Research and Review*, and *Endocrine*. He is the author of two books four book chapters, and the editor of four books. He has written 15 scripts for students, is the ad hoc reviewer of more than 30 peer-reviewed journals, and an editorial member of peer-reviewed journals. His research focuses on cells, physiology, genetics, and pathophysiology.

Editor of Volume 4: Leszek Szablewski
Medical University of Warsaw,
Warsaw, Poland

Book Series Editor: Angel Catala
National University of La Plata, Argentina

Scope of the Series

Modern physiology requires a comprehensive understanding of the integration of tissues and organs throughout the mammalian body, including the expression, structure, and function of molecular and cellular components. While a daunting task, learning is facilitated by our identification of common, effective signaling pathways employed by nature to sustain life. As a main example, the cellular interplay between intracellular Ca2 increases and changes in plasma membrane potential is integral to coordinating blood flow, governing the exocytosis of neurotransmitters and modulating genetic expression. Further, in this manner, understanding the systemic interplay between the cardiovascular and nervous systems has now become more important than ever as human populations age and mechanisms of cellular oxidative signaling are utilized for sustaining life. Altogether, physiological research enables our identification of clear and precise points of transition from health to development of multi-morbidity during the inevitable aging process (e.g., diabetes, hypertension, chronic kidney disease, heart failure, age-related macular degeneration; cancer). With consideration of all organ systems (e.g., brain, heart, lung, liver; gut, kidney, eye) and the interactions thereof, this Physiology Series will address aims of resolve (1) Aging physiology and progress of chronic diseases (2) Examination of key cellular pathways as they relate to calcium, oxidative stress, and electrical signaling & (3) how changes in plasma membrane produced by lipid peroxidation products affects aging physiology

Contents

Preface

Adipose Tissue—An Update is an update to the first volume, which was published by IntechOpen in 2018, and a part of the book series "Physiology." The chapters include information on adipose tissue such as the characterization of this tissue, the role of sirtuins in its metabolism, and its role in diseases. The book also includes a description of adipose tissue as an endocrine organ, as well as a signaling system in this tissue. This book is an important source of information because it describes several aspects of adipose tissue. Based on the interest of readers, IntechOpen decided to continue the publication of books on adipose tissue. Therefore, *Adipose Tissue—An Update* is the result of this continuation.

Adipose tissue is a kind of specialized connective tissue. Depending on its type, adipose tissue plays different and significant roles in humans and animals. For example, brown adipose tissue, which is found in fetuses and newborn, in adult humans is practically absent; in mammals it is involved in the process of thermogenesis, metabolizing fatty acids. White adipose tissue has different functions. It protects against environmental factors that can cause mechanical injury and cold. Other functions include the storage of lipids and triacylglycerol and the synthesis of fatty acids. During fasting, fatty acids are released and in the process of β-oxidation are a source of adenosine triphosphate. White adipose tissue is also a major secretory organ. White adipose tissue secretes bioactive molecules such as cholesterol, retinol, steroid hormones, prostaglandins, and proteins known as "adipokines" that influence human physiology and pathology. These molecules have a beneficial role. Unfortunately, they may also be associated with pathologies and diseases such as obesity and insulin resistance. They may increase the risk of metabolic syndrome, cardiovascular diseases, and others. Obesity, due to visceral accumulation of adipose tissue, is especially dangerous. It is suggested that release of fatty acids from the visceral depot into the portal vein increases gluconeogenesis and hepatic glucose output, causing insulin resistance. Insulin resistance, on the other hand, may cause type 2 diabetes mellitus. The World Health Organization defined type 2 diabetes mellitus as "a progressive worldwide epidemic." Visceral abdominal obesity reduces life expectancy by about 8 years. Beige adipose tissue histologically is similar to brown adipose tissue. Stimuli, such as cold, exercise, or thyroid hormones, cause differentiation of white adipose tissue into brown adipose tissue. This process is an adaptive and reversible response of white adipose tissue to stimuli.

In the past several decades, knowledge of adipose tissue has been rapidly growing. This book aims to provide an overview of the topics of adipose tissue and its role in human physiology and pathology. The book is written by authors from different laboratories, yet the editor has tried to arrange the chapters in an issue order to make it easier for readers to find what they need. The authors discuss adipose tissue from different aspects and hope to enhance a clear understanding of this histological, physiological, and pathological problem.

This book contains three sections focusing on the topic of adipose tissue. Section 1 contains only one chapter and presents the general characteristics of adipose tissue. Section 2, which includes Chapters 2–4, mainly describes the role of sirtuins, follistatin, and alcohol in the metabolism of adipose tissue. Finally, Section 3, which includes Chapters 5–7, focuses on the disorders in adipose tissue and their influence on human health and diseases.

I hope that this book will be of help to scientists, doctors, pharmacists, and other experts in various disciplines. It should also be suitable for teaching.

I would like to thank Ms. Marina Dusevic for her great effort in book planning and editing during the process of book publication.

dr. hab. Leszek Szablewski
Professor,
Medical University of Warsaw,
Warsaw, Poland

Section 1

General Characteristics of Adipose Tissue

Chapter 1

Introductory Chapter: Adipose Tissue

Leszek Szablewski

1. Introduction

Adipose tissue is a kind of connective tissue. It is a highly specialized tissue that plays a significant role in humans and animals. Adipocytes, cells of adipose tissue, store lipids and triacylglycerol as well as synthesize fatty acids. It also protects against mechanical injury as well as against cold. Adipose tissue is also involved in process of thermogenesis. Adipose tissue is also a metabolic active organ. Adipose tissue, beside adipocytes, contains also the stromal vascular fraction (SVF) of cells including fibroblasts, vascular endothelial cells, and immune cells, for example, macrophages.

2. Types of adipose tissue

Based on colors, adipose tissue is classified as white adipose tissue (WAT) and brown adipose tissue (BAT). These two types of adipocytes arise from separate progenitor cell lines. They show distinct morphology, structure, localization in the body, and function [1, 2].

White adipocytes are globular cells. Their size varies between 25 and 200 μm and depends on the size of the single lipid droplet accumulated within them [3, 4]. They contain large, single lipid droplet, more than 90% of the cell volume. Therefore, the amount of cytoplasm is small, and the nucleus is decentralized [5] and has a low density of mitochondria [3, 4]. Their main function is to store lipids, as energetic molecules to provide energy to the cells between the meals. White adipose tissue secretes also several molecules, such as retinol, steroid, hormones, prostaglandins, and adipokines that are pro- and anti-inflammatory cytokines. These molecules influence human and animal physiology and pathology.

White adipose tissue may be differentiated based on the anatomical locations or depots: subcutaneous (under the skin in the hypodermis region) and visceral. Increased visceral fat increases the risk of metabolic and cardiovascular diseases [6, 7]. Subcutaneous fat may protect against metabolic derangements [8]. Two subcutaneous fat regions in humans are recognized: upper and lower body fat. Accumulation of fat in lower regions (around the gluteal and femoral, the so-called gluteofemoral regions) improves glucose tolerance [9], negatively correlates with insulin resistance [8], and is associated with reduced aortic calcification [10]. Visceral adipose tissue is generally regarded as intra-abdominal adipose tissue. Visceral fat surrounds the internal organs. The major visceral depots are the omental, retroperitoneal, perineal, mesenteric, and pericardial depots [11, 12]. The mesenteric and omental adipose tissues drain directly into the portal circulation. These adipocytes release free fatty acids and pro-inflammatory cytokines to the liver. This process causes the development of hepatic steatosis and insulin resistance

[13, 14]. Pericardial fat increases the risk of metabolic disorders and low-grade inflammation, involved in type 2 diabetes and cardiac complication. It may cause also increased diastolic pressure and fasting insulin levels [15, 16] and arterial calcium accumulation [17] and severity of coronary disease [18]. Increased perirenal and pararenal depots are associated with glomerulopathy [19], chronic kidney diseases in patients with type 2 diabetes [20], and hypertension [21, 22]. Increased thickness of mesenteric fat is correlated with increased risk of cardiovascular diseases [23], Crohn's disease [24], hepatic insulin resistance, and hepatosteatosis [25]. These observations suggest that increased visceral fat deposition is associated with diseases and metabolic derangements, whereas subcutaneous fat deposition is not so dangerous.

Brown adipose tissues have polygonal shape, and their diameter is variable. They are smaller in comparison to WAT (15–60 μm) [26]. They also contain lipid droplets, but as multiple, small vacuoles of varied size. These cells contain a large amount of cytoplasm and centralized nucleus [5]. The most characteristic organelles presented in brown adipocytes are the mitochondria [27, 28]. BAT is found in fetuses and newborn, whereas in adult humans is practically absent. It is present at discrete sites such as in the upper trunk [29].

Recently, the third type of adipose tissue has been described. It is termed "brown-in-white," "brite," or "beige" [26, 30]. Beige adipose tissue histologically is very similar to BAT. The development of beige AT is due to the browning of WAT. It is an adaptive response to stimulation, for example, cold exposure, exercise, natriuretic peptides, thyroid hormones, bile acids, and so on [31–33]. Beige AT exhibits several intermediate features between BAT and WAT. For example, its adipocytes have a predominant lipid vacuole in the cytoplasm and numerous mitochondria [27, 34]. They express genes involved in the process of thermogenesis [30, 32, 33]. On the other hand, adipocytes of beige AT express characteristic and distinct gene markers. These gene markers are specific for beige adipocytes and distinguish them from adipocytes of BAT and WAT [26, 30, 35, 36].

3. Adipose tissue as an endocrine organ

As mentioned earlier, adipose tissue is also an endocrine organ. It secretes several hormones that regulate the homeostasis. The first molecule with hormonal activity secreted by adipocytes was leptin. It is a satiety hormone that suppresses food intake and increases energy expenditure. The levels of leptin are positively correlated with the amount of body fat [37]. Subcutaneous white adipose tissue secretes greater amounts of leptin than visceral WAT [38, 39]. Adiponectin, another hormone secreted by adipose tissue, is secreted primarily by subcutaneous rather than visceral fat. It shows anti-inflammatory and insulin-sensitizing roles [40]. In obese humans and patients with insulin resistance, the level of adiponectin is low [41, 42]. Resistin, a peptide hormone, impairs glucose and insulin metabolism and is implicated in insulin resistance [43, 44]. Visfatin is a hormone implicated in the utilization of glucose, predominantly synthesized and secreted in visceral fat [45]; however, it is predominantly secreted from macrophages rather than adipocytes. It has endocrine, paracrine, and autocrine functions and can bind to insulin receptor. There are also other hormones synthesized and secreted by adipose tissue such as acylation-stimulating protein (ASP) which is concerned with fat storage.

Adipose tissue secretes also growth factors, such as fibroblast growth factors (FGFs), insulin-like growth factor-1 (IGF-1), hepatocyte growth factor (HGF), nerve growth factor (NGF), vascular endothelial growth factor (VEGF), and transforming growth factor (TGF). These growth factors stimulate several processes such as adipogenesis [46], glucose metabolism [47], angiogenesis [48, 49], and thermogenesis [50]. On the other hand, some of these growth factors may be a pro-inflammatory adipokines. Adipose tissue secretes also other inflammatory cytokines such as interleukin-6, interleukin-8, interferon-γ, plasminogen activation inhibitor-1 as well as anti-inflammatory adipokines, such as adiponectin [51]. There are also many other molecules secreted by adipose tissue, such as retinol-binding protein 4 (RBP4), vaspin, omentin, chemerin, serum amyloid A (SAA), angiotensinogen, macrophage migration inhibitory factor (MIF), lipoprotein lipase, cholesterol ester transfer protein (CETP), prostaglandins, estrogens, glucocorticoids, and so on. All of these molecules influence human and animal processes. They have positive, as well as negative, effects on human health. Adipose tissue may be involved in the development of many diseases, such as type 2 diabetes mellitus [52, 53], metabolic syndrome [54], and several cancers (breast [55], cervical [56], endometrial [57], kidney [58], and gastrointestinal [59, 60]). Disturbances in functions of adipose tissue may cause also psychiatric diseases and disorders, such as depression [61], dementia [62], insomnia [63], and many others.

Author details

Leszek Szablewski
Medical University of Warsaw, Warsaw, Poland

*Address all correspondence to: leszek.szablewski@wum.edu.pl

References

[1] Scheja L, Heeren J. Metabolic interplay between white, beige, brown adipocytes and the liver. Journal of Hepatology. 2016;**64**:1176-1186

[2] Gaggini M, Carli F, Gastaldelli A. The color of fat and its central role in the development and progression of metabolic diseases. Hormone Molecular Biology and Clinical Investigation. 2017;**31**:1-14

[3] Schosserer M, Grillari J, Wolfrum C, Scheidler M. Age-induced changes in white, brite, and brown adipose depots: A mini-review. Gerontology. 2018;**64**:229-236

[4] Mathew H, Castracane VD, Mantzoros C. Adipose tissue and reproductive health. Metabolism. 2018;**86**:18-32

[5] Cinti S. The role of brown adipose tissue in human obesity. Nutrition, Metabolism, and Cardiovascular Diseases. 2006;**16**:569-574

[6] Gastaldeli A, Miyazaki Y, Pettiti M, Matsuda M, Mahankali S, Santini E, et al. Metabolic effects of visceral fat accumulation in type 2 diabetes. The Journal of Clinical Endocrinology and Metabolism. 2002;**87**:5098-5103

[7] Kissebah AH, Vydelingum N, Murray R, Evans DJ, Hartz AJ, Kalkhoff RK, et al. Relation of body fat distribution to metabolic complications of obesity. The Journal of Clinical Endocrinology and Metabolism. 1982;**54**:254-260

[8] Zhang M, Hu T, Zhang S, Zhou L. Associations of different adipose tissue depots with insulin resistance: A systemic review and meta-analysis of observational studies. Scientific Reports. 2015;**5**:18495

[9] Snijder MB, Dekker JM, Visser M, Yudkin JS, Stehouwer CD, Bouter LM, et al. Larger thigh and hip circumferences are associated with better glucose tolerance: The hoorn study. Obesity Research. 2003;**11**:104-111

[10] Tanko LB, Bagger YZ, Alexandersen P, Larsen PJ, Christiansen C. Peripheral adiposity exhibits an independent dominant antiatherogenic effect in elderly women. Circulation. 2003;**107**:1626-1631

[11] Cinti S. The adipose organ at a glance. Disease Models & Mechanisms. 2012;**5**:588-594

[12] Chusyd DE, Wang D, Huffman DM, Nagy TR. Relationships between rodent white adipose fat pads and human white adipose fat depots. Fronties in Nutrition. 2016;**63**:10

[13] Tchkonia T, Thomou T, Zhu Y, Karagiannides I, Pothoulakis C, Jensen MD, et al. Mechanisms and metabolic implications of regional differences among fat depots. Cell Metabolism. 2013;**17**:644-656

[14] Sackmann-Sala L, Berryman DE, Munn RD, Lubbers ER, Kopchick JJ. Heterogeneity among white adipose tissue depots in male C57BL/6J mice. Obesity (Silver Spring). 2012;**20**:101-111

[15] Fernández Muñoz MJ, Basurto Acevedo L, Córdova Pérez N, Vázquez Martínez AL, Tepach Gutiérrez N, Vega García S, et al. Epicardial adipose tissue is associated with visceral fat, metabolic syndrome, and insulin resistance in menopausal women. Revista Española de Cardiología (English Edition). 2014;**67**:436-441

[16] Iacobellis G, Ribaudo MC, Assael F, Vecci E, Tiberti C, Zappaterreno A, et al. Echocardiographic epicardial adipose tissue is related to anthropometric and clinical parameters

of metabolic syndrome: A new indicator of cardiovascular risk. The Journal of Clinical Endocrinology and Metabolism. 2003;**88**:5163-5168

[17] Rosito GA, Massaro JM, Hoffmann U, Ruberg FL, Mahabadi AA, Vasan RS, et al. Pericardial fat, visceral abdominal fat, cardiovascular disease risk factors and vascular calcification in a community-based sample: The Framingham Heart Study. Circulation. 2008;**117**:605-613

[18] Meenakshi K, Rajendran M, Srikumar S, Chidambaram S. Epicardial fat thickness: A surrogate marker of coronary artery disease—Assessment by echocardiography. Indian Heart Journal. 2016;**68**:336-341

[19] Cignarelli M, Lamacchia O. Obesity and kidney disease. Nutrition, Metabolism, and Cardiovascular Diseases. 2007;**17**:757-762

[20] Lamacchia O, Nicastro V, Camarchio D, Valente U, Grisorio R, Gesualdo L, et al. Para- and perirenal fat thickness is an independent predictor of chronic kidney disease, increased renal resistance index and hyperuricaemia in type-2 diabetic patients. Nephrology, Dialysis, Transplantation. 2011;**26**:892-898

[21] Chughtai HL, Morgan TM, Rocco M, Stacey B, Brinkley TE, Ding J, et al. Renal sinus fat and poor blood pressure control in middle-aged and elderly individuals at risk for cardiovascular events. Hypertension. 2010;**56**:901-906

[22] Ritz E, Koleganova N. Obesity and chronic kidney disease. Seminars in Nephrology. 2009;**29**:504-511

[23] Liu KH, Chan YL, Chan WB, Kong WL, Kong MO, Chan JC. Sonographic measurement of mesenteric fat thickness is a good correlate with cardiovascular risk factors. Comparison with subcutaneous and preperitoneal fat thickness, magnetic resonance imaging and anthropometric indexes. International Journal of Obesity and Related Metabolic Disorders. 2003;**27**:1267-1273

[24] Peyerin-Biroulet L, Gonzalez F, Dubuquoy L, Rousseaux C, Dubuquoy C, Decourcelle C, et al. Mesenteric fat as a source of C reactive protein and as a target for bacterial translocation in Crohn's disease. Gut. 2012;**61**:78-85

[25] Wueest RR, Item F, Lucchini FC, Challa TD, Müller W, Blüher M, et al. Mesenteric fat lipolysis mediates obesity-associated hepatic steatosis and insulin resistance. Diabetes. 2016;**65**:140-148

[26] Jeanson Y, Carrière A, Casteilla L. A new role for browning as a redox and stress adaptive mechanism? Frontiers in Endocrinology (Lausanne). 2015;**6**:158

[27] Cinti S. Transdifferentiation properties of adipocytes in the adipose organ. American Journal of Physiology. Endocrinology and Metabolism. 2009;**297**:E977-E986

[28] Saely CH, Geiger K, Drexel H. Brown versus white adipose tissue: A mini-review. Gerontology. 2012;**58**:15-23

[29] Giralt M, Villarroya F. White, brown, beige/brite: Different adipose cells for different functions? Endocrinology. 2013;**154**:2992-3000

[30] Vargas-Castillo A, Fuentes-Romero R, Rodriguez-Lopez LA, Torres N, Tovar AR. Understanding the biology of thermogenic fat: Is browning a new approach to the treatment of obesity? Archives of Medical Research. 2017;**48**:401-413

[31] Azhar Y, Parmar A, Miller CN, Samuels JS, Ryalam S. Phytochemicals as novel agents for the induction of browning in white adipose tissue.

Nutrition & Metabolism (London). 2016;**13**:89

[32] Castro É, Silva TEO, Festuccia WT. Critical review of beige adipocyte thermogenic activation and contribution to whole-body energy expenditure. Hormone Molecular Biology and Clinical Investigation. 2017;**31**(2)

[33] Stanford KI, Goodyear LJ. Exercise regulation of adipose tissue. Adipocytes. 2016;**5**:153-162

[34] Aldiss P, Betts J, Sale C, Pope M, Symonds ME. Exercise-induced "browning" of adipose tissues. Metabolism. 2018;**81**:63-70

[35] Waldén TB, Hansen IR, Timmons JA, Cannon B, Nedergaard J. Recruited vs. nonrecruited molecular signatures of brown, "brite", and white adipose tissues. American Journal of Physiology. Endocrinology and Metabolism. 2012;**302**:E19-E31

[36] Wu J, Boström P, Sparks LM, Ye L, Hoi JH, et al. Beige adipocytes are a distinct type of thermogenic fat cell in mouse and man. Cell. 2012;**150**:366-376

[37] Bastard JP, Maachi M, Lagathu C, Kim MJ, Caron M, Vidal H, et al. Recent advances in the relationship between obesity, inflammation, and insulin resistance. European Cytokine Network. 2006;**17**:4-12

[38] Atzmon G, Yang XM, Muzumdar R, Ma XH, Gabriely I, Barzilai N. Differential gene expression between visceral and subcutaneous fat depots. Hormone and Metabolic Research. 2002;**34**:622-628

[39] Montague CT, Prins JB, Sanders L, Zhang J, Sewter CP, Digby J, et al. Depot-related gene expression in human subcutaneous and omental adipocytes. Diabetes. 1998;**47**:1384-1391

[40] Fain JN, Madan AK, Hiler ML, Cheema P, Bahouth SW. Comparison of the release of adipokines by adipose tissue, adipose tissue matrix, and adipocytes from visceral and subcutaneous abdominal adipose tissues of obese humans. Endocrinology. 2004;**145**:2273-2282

[41] Lafontan M, Girard J. Impact of visceral adipose tissue on liver metabolism. Part I: Heterogenity of adipose tissue and functional properties of visceral adipose tissue. Diabetes & Metabolism. 2008;**34**(4 Pt 1):317-327

[42] Lihn AS, Bruun JM, He G, Pedersen SB, Jensen PF, Richelsen B. Lower expression of adiponectin mRNA in visceral adipose tissue in lean and obese subjects. Molecular and Cellular Endocrinology. 2004;**219**:9-15

[43] Steppan CM, Bailey ST, Bhat S, Brown EJ, Banerjee RR, Wright CM, et al. The hormone resistin links obesity to diabetes. Nature. 2001;**409**:307-312

[44] Muse ED, Obici S, Bhanot S, Monia BP, McKay RA, Rajala MW, et al. Role of resistin in diet-induced hepatic insulin resistance. The Journal of Clinical Investigation. 2004;**114**:232-239

[45] Fukuhara A, , Matsuda M, Nishizawa M, Segawa K, Tanaka M, Kishimoto K, et al. Visfatin: A protein secreted by visceral fat that mimics the effects of insulin. Science. 2005;**307**:426-430

[46] Mejhert N, Galitzky J, Pettersson AT, Bambace C, Blomqvist L, Boulomié A, et al. Mapping of the fibroblast growth factors in human white adipose tissue. The Journal of Clinical Endocrinology and Metabolism. 2010;**95**:2451-2457

[47] Entingh A, Kahn R. Differential roles of the insulin and insulin-like growth factor-1 (EGF-1) receptors

in response to insulin and IGF-1. The Journal of Biological Chemistry. 2004;**279**:38016-38024

[48] Mick GJ, Wang X, McCormick K. White adipocyte vascular endothelial growth factor: Regulation by insulin. Endocrinology. 2002;**143**:948-953

[49] Bell LN, Ward JL, Degawa M, Bovenkerk J, Jones R, Cacucci B, et al. Adipose tissue production of hepatocyte growth factor contributes to elevated serum HGF in obesity. American Journal of Physiology. Endocrinology and Metabolism. 2006;**291**:E843-E848

[50] Nisoli E, Tonello C, Benarese M, Liberini P, Carruba MO. Expression of nerve growth factor in brown adipose tissue: Implications for thermogenesis and obesity. Endocrinology. 1996;**137**:495-503

[51] DeFuria J, Belkina AC, Jagannathan-Bogdan M, Snyder-Cappione J, Carr JD, Nersesova YR, et al. B cells promote inflammation in obesity and type 2 diabetes through regulation of T-cell function and an inflammatory cytokine profile. Proceedings of the National Academy of Sciences of the United States of America. 2013;**110**:5133-5138

[52] Fantuzzi G. Adipose tissue, adipokines, and inflammation. Journal of Allergy and Clinical Immunology. 2005;**115**:911-919

[53] Akash MSH, Rehman K, Liaqat A. Tumor necrosis factor-alpha: Role in development of insulin resistance and pathogenesis of type 2 diabetes mellitus. Journal of Cellular Biochemistry. 2018;**119**:105-110

[54] Mauvais-Jarvis F, Clegg DJ, Hevener AL. The role of estrogens in control of energy balance and glucose homeostasis. Endocrine Reviews. 2013;**34**:309-338

[55] White AJ, Nichols HB, Bradshaw PT, Sandler DP. Overall and central adiposity and breast cancer risk in the sister study. Cancer. 2015;**121**:3700-3708

[56] Poorolajal J, Jenabi E. The association between BMI and cervical cancer risk: A meta-analysis. European Journal of Cancer Prevention. 2016;**25**:232-238

[57] Plaza-Parrochia F, Romero C, Valladares L, Vega M. Endometrium and steroids, a pathologic overview. Steroids. 2017;**126**:85-91

[58] Kovesdy CP, Furth SL, Zoccali C. Obesity and kidney disease: Hidden consequence of the epidemic. Future Science Open Access. 2017;**3**:Fso159

[59] Chen Y, Liu L, Wang X. Body mass index and risk of gastric cancer: A meta-analysis of a population with more than ten million from 24 prospective studies. Cancer Epidemiology, Biomarkers and Prevention. 2013;**22**:1395-1408

[60] Ning Y, Wang L, Giovannucci EL. A quantitative analysis of body mass index and colorectal cancer: Finding from 56 observational studies. Obesity Reviews. 2010;**11**:19-30

[61] Thormann J, Chittka T, Minkwitz J, Kluge M, Himmerich H. Obesity and depression: An overview on the complex interactions of two diseases. Fortschritte der Neurologie-Psychiatrie. 2013;**81**:145-153

[62] Yaffe K, Falvey C, Harris TB, Newman A, Satterfield S, Koster A, et al. Effect of socioeconomic disparities on incidence of dementia among biracial older adults: Prospective study. British Medical Journal. 2013;**347**:f7051

[63] Buysse DJ. Insomnia. Journal of the American Medical Association. 2013;**309**:706-716

Section 2

Physiology of Adipose Tissue

Chapter 2

Role of Sirtuins in Adipose Tissue Development and Metabolism

Alina Kurylowicz

Abstract

Sirtuins (silent information regulators, sirts) via modification of histones, as well as transcription factors and co-regulators, control expression of other genes, particularly those involved in the organism response to stress. Detection of sirtuin expression in adipocytes initiated interest in their role in adipose tissue development and metabolism. This chapter presents how sirtuins control the critical steps of preadipocytes' differentiation and proliferation, as well as the process of adipose tissue browning. Moreover, it shows in vitro and in vivo data proving that sirtuins are involved in the regulation of lipogenesis, lipolysis, and secretory activity of adipose tissue. Due to all these reasons, sirtuins may constitute potential targets in the treatment of obesity and related complications.

Keywords: sirtuins, adipocytes, adipogenesis, lipid metabolism, adipokines

1. Introduction

Recent research widened our understanding of the role of adipose tissue from the simple energy storage to the metabolically and hormonally active organ that in response to environmental stimuli is able not only to activate lipolysis/lipogenesis but also to secrete several factors to communicate with and regulate the function of other organs. These findings allowed to understand the link between excess adiposity and the development of obesity-related complications and renewed interest in adipose tissue as a possible target for obesity-orientated therapies [1].

However, despite the constant progress in understanding its pathogenesis, the therapeutic potential to prevent and combat obesity is limited. Behavioral interventions, calorie restriction (CR) combined with the increased physical activity, do not assure persistent, long-term effects, while available pharmacological treatments allow for loss of 5–10% of initial weight. Therefore, there is a need for novel methods of treatment of obesity and its complications.

Studies on the influence of CR on the whole body function allow to identify sirtuins (silent information regulators, sirts)—essential players in different cellular metabolic pathways that seem to be crucial for the proper function of adipose tissue and in this way may constitute attractive therapeutic targets in the treatment of obesity and related complications.

2. A short review of the sirt system

The sirts are highly conserved regulatory proteins present almost in all species. Initially, they have been identified as class III histone deacetylases, nicotinamide adenine dinucleotide (NAD)-dependent enzymes responsible for the removal of acetyl groups from lysine residues in proteins, while some members of this family act also as mono-ADP-ribosyltransferases. Since acetylation and deacetylation are essential mechanisms of posttranslational modifications of proteins determining their activity, sirts were found to be involved in the regulation of distinct cellular pathways including, among others, those related to cell survival, apoptosis, inflammatory and stress responses, as well as lipid and glucose homeostases [2].

In human, seven sirt genes (*sirts*) have been identified that encode seven sirt enzymes of different structure, cellular localization, and tissue expression. All of them share a common conserved catalytic core region consisting of approximately 275 amino acids, forming a Rossmann fold domain (characteristic of NAD^+/NADH-binding proteins) and a zinc-binding domain connected by several loops [2]. Outside the catalytic core, sirt enzymes possess variable N- and C-terminal regions that decide about their enzymatic activities, binding partners and substrates, as well as subcellular localization [3]. sirt1, sirt6, and sirt7 localize predominantly in the nucleus where via modifications of transcription factors, cofactors, and histones they participate in the regulation of energy metabolism, stress and inflammatory responses, DNA repair (sirt1 and sirt6), and rDNA transcription (sirt7) [4]. sirt2 is a cytoplasmic sirtuin and plays a role in cell cycle control [5]. sirt3 can be found in mitochondria where it takes part in the regulation of enzymes involved, e.g., in glycolysis, fatty acid (FA) oxidation, ketone body synthesis, and the catabolism of amino acids as well as of apoptosis and oxidative stress pathways. This sirtuin also has as a nuclear full-length form (FL-sirt3) that is processed to the short mitochondrial form. Therefore, sirt3 may regulate cellular metabolism both at the transcriptional and posttranscriptional levels. sirt4 is also localized in mitochondria and acts as ADP-ribosylase. Another mitochondrial sirtuin—sirt5—has a potent demalonylation and desuccinylation enzymatic activity and is involved in the regulation of amino acid catabolism [6]. Importantly, the subcellular localization of sirts may vary in different cell types and may depend on their molecular interactions as it was shown in the case of sirt1, sirt2, and sirt3 that can be found both in the nucleus and in the cytoplasm [4].

Expression of *sirts* was detected in various human tissues, including those crucial for the regulation of metabolism, e.g., hypothalamus, liver, pancreatic islets, skeletal muscles, and adipocytes [7–10]. In these tissues, sirts control the expression of other genes, particularly those involved in the organism response to stress. It was shown that *sirt* expression and activity of sirt enzymes are highly sensitive to several environmental factors, CR, exercise, and cold exposure that represents an adaptive mechanism in response to environmental stress [3]. Fluctuations in intracellular NAD+ levels in response to nutrient availability are believed to mediate in this phenomenon. When nutrients are plentiful, cellular metabolism relies on glycolysis to produce energy, leading to the generation of ATP and conversion of NAD^+ to NADH. Low levels of NAD^+ and high levels of NADH result in inactivation of the enzymatic activity of sirts. In turn CR leads to the elevation of NAD+ levels in most metabolically active tissues resulting in the increased sirt activity [11]. In humans, obesity leads to downregulation of sirt1 level in adipose tissue that can be restored by the weight loss [12].

3. sirts and adipogenesis

sirts are considered as potential targets for the treatment of obesity that results from their involvement in the regulation of adipogenesis and adipocyte browning.

3.1 Types of adipocytes

In mammals, there are two main types of adipose tissue that differ in their structure, physiology, and function. White adipose tissue (WAT) acts mainly as energy storage that releases FA for the production of adenosine triphosphate (ATP) during the process of β-oxidation.

Small mammals and human newborns, apart from white adipocytes, possess large deposits of brown adipose tissue (BAT) responsible for the non-shivering (adaptive) thermogenesis which is for them the most important regulatory mechanism for maintaining body temperature. The energy produced due to the oxidation of lipolysis-derived FA in the BAT mitochondria is released as heat, mostly thanks to uncoupling proteins (UCP). Age progression in humans was believed to be associated with complete atrophy of BAT; however, novel methods of imaging led to the identification of BAT stores in several areas of the adult human body, as well as of cells reminding brown adipocytes dispersed within WAT also known as beige/brite adipocytes (BeAT). These cells share common morphological features of white and brown adipocytes, and their number may increase upon different stimuli (e.g., cold, exercise, thyroid hormones, resveratrol). There are two theories regarding BeAT origin: they (i) differentiate from the progenitor cells resident in WAT or (ii) arise due to the transdifferentiation of white adipocytes. Given the role of adaptive thermogenesis in the whole body energy expenditure, stimulation of white adipocytes browning seems to be an attractive therapeutic pathway in the treatment of obesity and related metabolic disorders [13].

3.2 sirts and preadipocyte differentiation

Peroxisome proliferator-activated receptor γ (PPARγ) is considered to be the main transcription factor responsible for promoting adipogenesis. sirt1, by interacting with two PPARγ corepressors, nuclear receptor corepressor (N-CoR) and silencing mediator of retinoid and thyroid hormone receptors (SMRT), can attenuate adipogenesis [14]. Consistently, overexpression of ectopic *sirt1* blocks adipogenesis in 3T3-L1 cells, a culture of mouse adipocytes used as a model of adipocyte differentiation [15, 16]. Additionally, via activation of the Wnt signaling pathway, sirt1 determinates mesenchymal stem cells (MSC) differentiation toward myogenic cells, while its inhibition in MSC promotes adipogenesis [17]. MicroRNA 146b (miR-146b) acts as a negative regulator of sirt1 during adipocyte differentiation, giving a hope that interference with this miRNA may constitute a therapeutic perspective in the treatment of excess adiposity [18].

Another sirtuin family member—sirt2—has also shown an inhibitory effect on adipocyte differentiation [14]. In this process, sirt2 deacetylates forkhead box O1 (FOXO1) transcription factor and subsequently represses PPARγ transcriptional activity [19]. Therefore, *sirt2* overexpression inhibits adipogenesis, while its silencing has an opposite effect in 3 T3-L1 preadipocytes. Moreover, this inhibitory influence of sirt2 on adipocyte differentiation discloses under CR that indicates the role of this sirtuin in the maintenance of energy homeostasis and suggests that sirt2 activators could provide novel therapeutics of obesity and its complications; however, such compounds have not been developed yet.

sirt3 is essential for the activation of bioenergetic function of mitochondria at the early stage of adipocyte differentiation. Silencing of sirt3 decreases the protein level of forkhead box O3a (FoxO3a) transcription factor and subsequently downregulates the expression of several antioxidant enzymes and increases oxidative stress in MSCs after adipogenic induction. In this way, sirt3 depletion diminishes the ability of MSCs to undergo adipogenic differentiation and leads to adipocyte dysfunction [20].

Knockout of *sirt4* (encoding sirt4) leads to the decreased expression of adipogenic differentiation marker genes during differentiation of bovine adipocytes, suggesting that this sirtuin is crucial for the proper adipogenesis too [21].

sirt6 and sirt7 were also found to be necessary for adipocyte differentiation, and their deficiency inhibits the development of preadipocytes toward white adipocytes. sirt6 inhibits the expression of kinesin family member 5C (KIF5C) and enhances casein kinase 2 (CK2) and in this way promotes mitotic clonal expansion of adipocytes [22]. Deletion of *sirt7* or inhibition of sirt7 diminishes the ability of mouse embryo fibroblasts and 3T3L1 cells to undergo adipogenesis. However, its overexpression did not rescue the preadipocyte differentiation, suggesting that sirt7 is required but not sufficient to perform a full program of adipogenesis. Interestingly, sirt7 is a metabolic target for miR-93, a negative regulator of adipogenesis, which expression is decreased in genetically obese ob/ob mice [23].

Experimental data suggest a direct interaction between sirt1 and sirt7 proteins at the molecular level as it was shown in immunoprecipitation assays and in vivo, where sirt7 knockout (KO) mice have increased sirt1 protein levels and enzymatic activity in WAT. Loss of sirt7 leads to increased sirt1 activity and recruitment to the PPARγ promoter, causing downregulation of its expression, that can explain the lipodystrophic phenotype in sirt7 KO mice [24].

The role of sirts in preadipocyte differentiation is schematically shown in **Figure 1**.

3.3 sirts and adipocyte browning

One of the approaches to the treatment of obesity is based on the activation in preadipocyte genes specific to BAT, which is characterized by high metabolic activity. Browning (brightening or beiging) of white adipocytes is an adaptive and reversible process that occurs in response to various stimuli.

Since sirt1, by direct deacetylation of PPARγ, recruits the BAT program coactivator Prdm16 (PR domain containing 16) to PPARγ, it also plays a crucial role

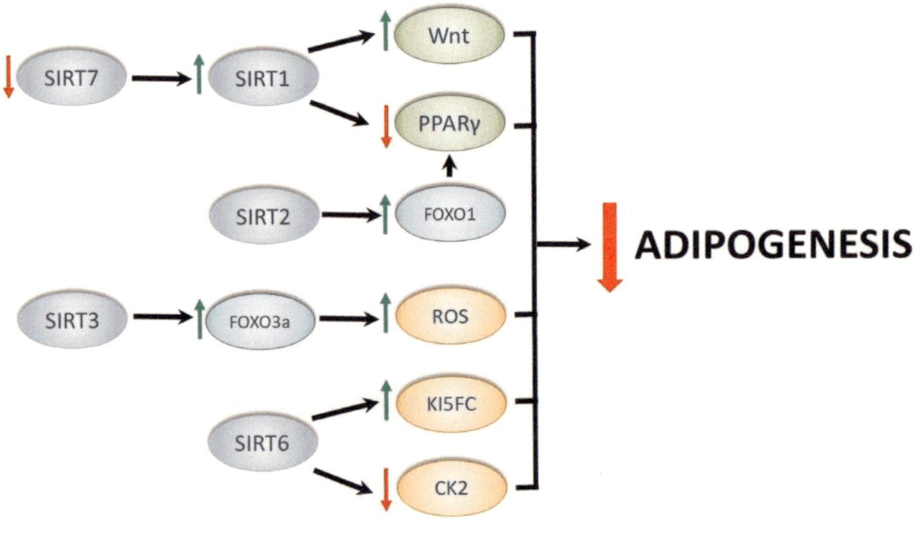

Figure 1.
Role of sirtuins in adipocyte differentiation. CK2, casein kinase 2; FOXO1, forkhead box O1; FOXO3a, forkhead box O3a; KI5FC, kinesin family member 5C; PPARγ, peroxisome proliferator-activated receptor γ; ROS, reactive oxygen species; sirt, sirtuin; Wnt, signaling pathway; ↑, upregulation and stimulation; ↓, downregulation and inhibition.

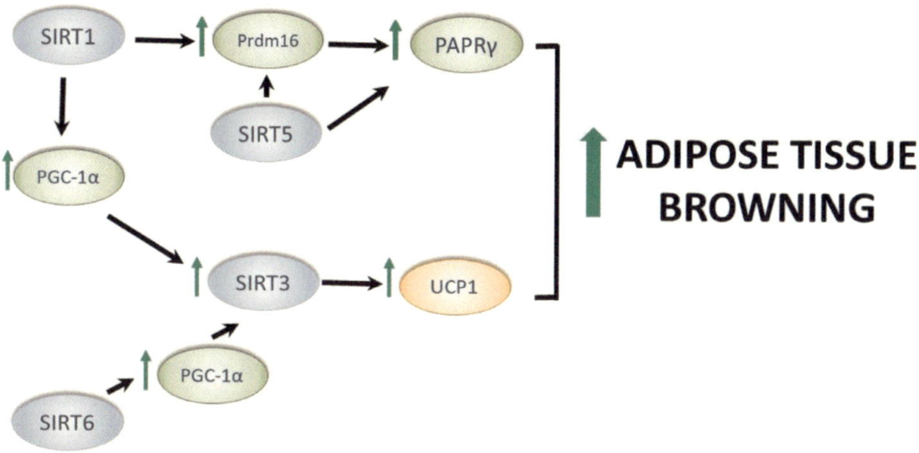

Figure 2.
Role of sirtuins in adipocyte browning. PGC-1α, PPARγ coactivator 1α; PPARγ, peroxisome proliferator-activated receptor γ; Prdm16, PR domain containing 16; sirt, sirtuin; UCP, uncoupling protein 1; ↑, upregulation and stimulation.

in the induction of genes typical for BAT and repression of WAT genes associated with insulin resistance [25]. Therefore, silencing of *sirt1* in 3T3-L1 preadipocytes leads to their hyperplasia and increased expression of WAT and inflammatory markers with a parallel decrease in BAT markers, whereas its activation results in increased adipocyte browning [26].

Cooperation among different sirtuins is crucial for the proper differentiation of brown adipocytes. For example, nutritional and thermal stress induces sirt1, which, by its deacetylation, activates PPARγ coactivator 1α (PGC-1α*)* which upregulates transcription of *sirt3*. In cultures of brown adipocyte precursors (HIB1B cells), overexpression of sirt3 resulted in the increased phosphorylation of the *cAMP response element-binding* protein (CREB) which then directly activates PGC-1α promoter, resulting in the increased expression of UCP1 and in promotion of mitochondrial respiration [27]. However, subsequent experiments showed that the protein produced based on the cDNA used in this experiment lacked proper deacetylase activity, so this finding should be treated with caution [28]. Moreover, sirt3 KO mice, despite mitochondrial protein hyperacetylation, showed no significant disturbances of the adaptive thermogenesis [29].

sirt5 was found to be essential for activation of brown adipogenic genes, and adipocyte differentiation in vitro and its knockout leads to the decrease in intracellular α-ketoglutarate concentration, which results in elevated histone methylation and transcriptional repression of *pparγ* and *Prdm16*. Therefore sirt5 KO mice present diminished browning capacity of WAT with subsequent cold intolerance [30].

Finally, depletion of sirt6 in primary brown adipocytes reduces binding of the activating transcription factor 2 (ATF2) to the PGC-1α promoter and in this way decreases basal mitochondrial respiration and maximal mitochondrial capacity [31].

The role of sirts in adipocyte browning is schematically shown in **Figure 2**.

4. sirts in control of adipose tissue function

Both in vitro and in vivo studies have implicated sirts in the regulation of adipose tissue metabolism. These studies let us understand the complexity of sirt actions and gave hope that the modulation of their activity may constitute a new therapeutic strategy for the treatment of obesity and its metabolic complications including hyperlipidemia and chronic inflammation.

4.1 sirts in lipid metabolism

sirts are expressed in tissues and organs involved in lipid metabolism including the liver, skeletal muscle, and white and brown adipose tissues, where they control lipid synthesis, storage, and utilization both directly and indirectly (via control of insulin secretion).

During fasting sirt1, by deacetylation of PPARγ corepressors (FOXO1 and PGC-*1α*), stimulates in the adipose tissue transcription of the gene encoding adipose triglyceride lipase (ATGL) and subsequent lipolysis. This process is impaired in sirt1 KO mice [15]. However, the results of animal studies regarding *sirt1* overexpression on body weight and composition are inconsistent [32, 33]. It is suggested that these discrepancies may be attributed to the different levels of *sirt1* expression between the transgenic animals as well as to the differences between strains and species used in the experiments.

Apart from the regulation of PPARα-related pathways, sirt1 may influence FA metabolism via downregulation of sterol regulatory element-binding proteins 1 and 2 (SREBP-1 and SREBP-2) transcription factors. sirt1 overexpression or its activation by, e.g., resveratrol (RSV), prevents cleavage-induced activation of SERBs and their translocation to the nucleus where they promote transcription of genes crucial for sterol biosynthesis [34]. sirt1 KO mice have lower SREBP-1 mRNA levels in the liver that correlates with decreased serum triglyceride concentrations [35]. Activation of sirt1 also induces phosphorylation of AMP-activated protein kinase (AMPK) that protects against FA synthase induction and lipid accumulation caused by high glucose [36].

sirt1 also promotes deacetylation of liver X receptor (LXR) proteins and transcription factors that act as cholesterol sensors and regulate whole body cholesterol and lipid homeostasis [37]. LXR deacetylation is necessary both for their activation and induction of LXR target genes and for their subsequent ubiquitination. sirt1 KO animals have reduced mRNA levels of LXR target genes that result in impaired reverse cholesterol transport—a process by which excess cholesterol is removed from the peripheral cells and transported to the liver where it can be converted to bile and excreted [38].

Fasting and cold exposure were found to increase the expression of sirt2 in WAT. That results in the deacetylation of FOXO1 and subsequent repression of PPARγ activity, lipolysis, and release of FA. Similar effect can be obtained by administration of isoproterenol that confirms the role of adrenergic signaling in the regulation of sirt2 expression in WAT [19]. sirt2 may also inhibit lipogenesis by deacetylation of ATP-citrate lyase (ACLY), an enzyme crucial for FA synthesis. A deacetylated form of ACLY is then ubiquitinated and degraded, while lipogenesis is reduced [39].

Livers from sirt3 KO mice showed higher levels of FA oxidation intermediate products and triglycerides during fasting that was associated with decreased levels of FA oxidation when compared to wild-type animals. These findings are consistent with the fact that deacetylation of the long-chain acyl-coenzyme A dehydrogenase by sirt3 was found to determine proper mitochondrial FA oxidation [40].

There are experimental data that other sirts are also involved in lipid metabolism: in adipose tissue, e.g., deacetylation of malonyl-CoA-decarboxylase by sirt4 and desuccinylation of the hydroxyl-coenzyme A dehydrogenase by sirt5 determine proper mitochondrial FA oxidation [41, 42], while downregulation of sirt4 level results in the increased expression of genes involved in FA oxidation [43]. In experimental animals, sirt6 deficiency leads to impaired lipolytic activity and subsequent adipocyte hypertrophy [44]. On the molecular level, sirt6 deficiency increases the acetylation and phosphorylation of FOXO1, leading to its nuclear exclusion and decrease in its transcriptional activity that downregulates the expression of the gene encoding ATGL [44]. In turn, sirt6 overexpression in adipose tissue counteracts lipotoxicity caused by the high-fat diet by decreasing PPARγ signaling and diacylglycerol acyltransferase 1 (DGAT1) activity [45]. The role of sirt7 in lipid metabolism is yet to be determined. In some studies sirt7 KO mice, due to the impaired management of the endoplasmic reticulum stress, have increased lipogenesis in the liver that results in liver steatosis and dyslipidemia [23], while sirt7 upregulation restores hepatic homeostasis in diet-induced obesity [46]. On the contrary, other researchers showed that sirt7 via inhibition of testicular receptor 4 (TR4) degradation promotes FA uptake, triglyceride biosynthesis, and storage [47].

These results constituted the basis for studies on the use of sirtuin-activating compounds in order to increase lipolysis and to prevent excess adiposity.

4.2 sirts in control of adipose tissue inflammation and secretory activity

Recent years widened our understanding of the role of WAT which is now considered not only an energy storage but also an important endocrine organ that via secreted mediators (e.g., cytokines and adipokines) may influence the function of the whole organism and be responsible for the development of obesity-related complications.

sirt1, by interference with the nuclear factor κB (NF-κB) signaling pathway, represses inflammatory gene expression in adipocytes and in macrophages infiltrating adipose tissue, which results in the improvement of insulin signaling and in the reduction of hyperinsulinemia accompanied by an increase in insulin sensitivity in vivo [48, 49]. sirt1 can inhibit NF-κB signaling both directly and indirectly. Acting directly sirt1 deacetylates the RelA/p65 subunit of the NF-κB, leading to its subsequent ubiquitination and degradation. Indirect inhibition of NF-κB by sirt1 takes place by increasing activity of repressive transcriptional complexes, e.g., PPARα, which can bind and inactivate RelA/p65 or increase expression of the gene encoding inhibitor α of κB (IκBα) [50].

Similarly, overexpression of sirt6 suppresses activation of the NF-κB signaling in cell lines, firstly, by the direct interaction with NF-κB subunit and, secondly, by deacetylation of histone H3 lysine 9 at target gene promoters leading to inhibition of the transcription of the proinflammatory genes [51]. Moreover, sirt6 by binding to the c-Jun downregulates expression of its target genes including interleukin 6 (IL-6), tumor necrosis factor α (TNF-α), and monocyte chemoattractant protein 1 (MCP-1) [52]. Subsequently, in model animals, sirt1 and sirt6 deficiency increases macrophage infiltration in adipose tissue and subsequent inflammation [44]. Moreover, sirt1 deficiency in adipocytes (probably due to the decreased expression of IL-4) led to the shift between the profiles of macrophages from the anti-inflammatory (M2) to the proinflammatory (M1) [53]. Therefore, sirt1- and sirt6-deficient adipocytes are more potent in promoting macrophages migration than wild-type cells that can be reversed by addition of MCP1 or adiponectin.

This last adipokine is a protein hormone with many desirable metabolic properties (including anti-inflammatory and anti-oxidative effects) almost exclusively produced in adipocytes. sirt1 tightly regulates the expression and secretion of adiponectin by adipocytes: enhancing formation of the complex between FOXO1 and C/EBPα (CCAAT/enhancer binding protein α) increases expression of the *ADIPOQ* gene, while inhibition of endoplasmic reticulum oxidoreductase Ero-Lα decreases secretion of the high-molecular-weight (HMW) adiponectin [54]. Omentin-1 (intelectin-1) is another adipokine secreted, but not only by adipose tissue with anti-inflammatory properties that via activation of sirt1 exert its molecular effects on target genes [55].

In contrary, resistin is a hormone with biological characteristics opposite to adiponectin and omentin. It is secreted, apart from other sites, by adipose tissue; however, resistin expression in isolated human adipocytes is low, and its content in adipose tissue is proportional to the intensity of macrophages infiltration, which are the primary source of this adipokine [56]. Stimulation of sirt1 by RSV reduces resistin mRNA level and protein expression in macrophages, whereas sirt1 KO results in the opposite effect. On the molecular level, sirt1 interacts directly with the resistin promoter region at an activator protein 1 (AP-1) transcription factor response element as well as inhibits transactivation of the resistin gene by c-Jun pathway [57]. In animal model RSV, via activation of sirt1 was also found to decrease expression of visfatin—another adipokine secreted by macrophages infiltrating adipose tissue [58].

5. Sirtuins as targets for obesity treatment

Given their role in the regulation of lipid metabolism, adipogenesis and secretory activity of adipose tissue sirts constitute promising targets for novel therapies, targeting excess adiposity and associated metabolic disorders. However, the discovery of a compound that would be able to activate some sirt isoforms and to inhibit others is still a challenge. Another obstacle is to obtain tissue specificity of action for these compounds, since sirt activity may depend on the cell type and environmental factors.

Several sirt isoforms bear the potential for being used as therapeutic targets, but to date, only modulators of sirt1 have entered into the clinic. The most effective sirtuin-activating compound able to increase sirt1 activity in vitro by >10 fold is RSV [59]. RSV, naturally present in grapes and red wine, successfully inhibited maturation of preadipocytes and induced adipocyte apoptosis in cell cultures [60]. When administered to mice on the high-calorie diet, RSV was able to improve their metabolic and inflammatory profiles [61]. A reformulated version of RSV (resVida) with improved bioavailability was effective in decreasing glucose and triglyceride levels, reducing the intensity of inflammation and liver steatosis in obese men [62]. Another micronized formulation of RSV, SRT501, via activation of the similar set of genes as in the case of CR, was able to counteract negative consequences of a high-calorie diet in mice [63]. A composition containing RSV, leucine, β-hydroxymethyl butyrate (HMB), and ketoisocaproic acid synergistically activating sirt1 and sirt3 can induce FA oxidation and mitochondrial biogenesis. This combination, when tested on 3LT3-L1 preadipocytes, was more effective in activation of sirt1 than RSV alone but also able to activate sirt3. In c57/BL6 mice, treatment with a combination of low doses of RSV with either HMB or leucine resulted in a reduction of body weight and improvement of body composition accompanied by increased insulin sensitivity [64].

A variety of synthetic RSV derivatives with lower toxicity and higher potency to activate sirt1 have been invented. The example of them is SRT1720, able to increase deacetylation of sirt1 substrates in vitro and successfully applied in vivo to treat insulin resistance in animal models of type 2 diabetes [63, 65, 66]. Apart from the favorable influence on glucose metabolism, SRT1720, by decreasing expression of lipogenic genes, occurred to be effective in the treatment of animal models of liver steatosis [67]. However, some studies question the beneficial effect of SRT1720 on metabolic parameters in animals fed a high-fat diet [68]. Moreover, RSV and other sirt1 activators (SRT1720, SRT2183, SRT1460) were found not to activate sirt1 directly but by the activation of AMPK that increases intracellular NAD^+ levels and in this way induces deacetylation of sirt1 targets [69]. However, studies on sirt1 mutations that influence the protein structure suggest that there is also a direct interaction of RSV derivates with the sirt1 enzyme molecule [64]. In humans, administration of SRT2104 (another RSV analogue) caused a decrease in serum total cholesterol and triglycerides levels as well as a significant reduction of the inflammatory response to *lipopolysaccharide* stimulation [70].

Despite their beneficial effects on adipose tissue metabolism, the critical issue that may arise during the use of sirt1 activators in everyday practice is their limited target specificity that might result in unexpected adverse effects [71]. That is why sirt modulators are still under consideration before they can be approved for the routine treatment of obesity and metabolic disorders.

Till now, the only aspects in which sirt inhibitors can be used to treat obesity-associated metabolic disorders are to induce favorable changes in body composition. sirt1-inhibiting compounds such as splitomycin, suramin, salermide, EX-527, or sirtinol can be used to increase the amount of skeletal muscle. This concept is based on animal studies where sirt1 KO mice display higher muscle growth than wild-type animals and mice with muscle-specific *sirt1* overexpression [64]. However, sirt1 inhibitors were not tested for that purpose in humans.

Recently there has been a rapidly growing interest in the role of miRNAs in fat cell development and obesity, and there is also evidence that miRNA plays a role in the regulation of sirt activity [18, 23, 46, 72]. Therefore, one can assume that strategies based on modifying the action of sirts by specific miRNAs may also be useful in treating obesity. However, these studies are still at a preliminary stage.

6. Final remarks and conclusions

If the remarkable effects of sirts on adipose tissue development and metabolism coming from animal studies hold up in humans, their activators and inhibitors may revolutionize the treatment of obesity and associated complications. However, one should remember that sirt activities are not limited to the regulation of metabolism and include, also, e.g., control of longevity, oncogenesis as well as the function of neural and cardiovascular systems. Therefore, compounds targeting sirts' system in order to combat excess adiposity have to be adipose tissue-specific to avoid potentially harmful and counterproductive side effects of global sirt activation/inactivation. Till now such compounds have not been accepted for the clinical practice; however, many of them are under evaluation, and it is very likely that shortly new therapeutic strategies aimed at selective and tissue-specific modulation of sirt activity will be registered for the treatment of obesity and its complications.

Author details

Alina Kurylowicz
Department of Human Epigenetics, Mossakowski Medical Research Centre, Polish Academy of Sciences, Warsaw, Poland

*Address all correspondence to: akurylowicz@imdik.pan.pl

References

[1] Galic S, Oakhill JS, Steinberg GR. Adipose tissue as an endocrine organ. Molecular and Cellular Endocrinology. 2010;**316**:129-139. DOI: 10.1016/j.mce.2009.08.018

[2] Sanders BD, Jackson B, Marmorstein R. Structural basis for sirtuin function: What we know and what we don't. Biochimica et Biophysica Acta. 2010;**1804**:1604-1616. DOI: 10.1016/j.bbapap.2009.09.009

[3] Haigis MC, Guarente LP. Mammalian sirtuins—Emerging roles in physiology, aging, and calorie restriction. Genes & Development. 2006;**20**:2913-2921. DOI: 10.1101/gad.1467506

[4] Haigis MC, Sinclair DA. Mammalian sirtuins: Biological insights and disease relevance. Annual Review of Pathology. 2010;**5**:253-295. DOI: 10.1146/annurev.pathol.4.110807.092250

[5] Wang F, Nguyen M, Qin FX, Tong Q. sirt2 deacetylates FOXO3a in response to oxidative stress and caloric restriction. Aging Cell. 2007;**6**:505-514. DOI: 10.1111/j.1474-9726.2007.00304.x

[6] Parihar P, Solanki I, Mansuri ML, Parihar MS. Mitochondrial sirtuins: Emerging roles in metabolic regulations, energy homeostasis and diseases. Experimental Gerontology. 2015;**61**:130-141. DOI: 10.1016/j.exger.2014.12.004

[7] Zakhary SM, Ayubcha D, Dileo JN, Jose R, Leheste JR, Horowitz JM, et al. Distribution analysis of deacetylase sirt1 in rodent and human nervous systems. The Anatomical Record. 2010;**293**:1024-1032. DOI: 10.1002/ar.21116

[8] Moschen AR, Wieser V, Gerner RR, Bichler A, Enrich B, Moser P, et al. Adipose tissue and liver expression of sirt1, 3, and 6 increase after extensive weight loss in morbid obesity. Journal of Hepatology. 2013;**59**:1315-1322. DOI: 10.1016/j.jhep.2013.07.027

[9] Caton PW, Richardson SJ, Kieswich J, Bugliani M, Holland ML, Marchetti P, et al. Sirtuin 3 regulates mouse pancreatic beta cell function and is suppressed in pancreatic islets isolated from human type 2 diabetic patients. Diabetologia. 2013;**56**:1068-1077. DOI: 10.1007/s00125-013-2851-y

[10] Acs Z, Bori Z, Takeda M, Osvath P, Berkes I, Taylor AW, et al. High altitude exposure alters gene expression levels of DNA repair enzymes, and modulates fatty acid metabolism by sirt4 induction in human skeletal muscle. Respiratory Physiology & Neurobiology. 2014;**196**:33-37. DOI: 10.1016/j.resp.2014.02.006

[11] Chalkiadaki A, Guarente L. Sirtuins mediate mammalian metabolic responses to nutrient availability. Nature Reviews Endocrinology. 2012;**8**:287-296. DOI: 10.1038/nrendo.2011.225

[12] Kurylowicz A, Owczarz M, Polosak J, Jonas MI, Lisik W, Jonas M, et al. sirt1 and sirt7 expression in adipose tissues of obese and normal-weight individuals is regulated by microRNAs but not by methylation status. International Journal of Obesity. 2016;**40**:1635-1642. DOI: 10.1038/ijo.2016.131

[13] Zwick RK, Guerrero-Juarez CF, Horsley V, Plikus MV. Anatomical, physiological, and functional diversity of adipose tissue. Cell Metabolism. 2018;**27**:68-83. DOI: 10.1016/j.cmet.2017.12.002

[14] Jing E, Gesta S, Kahn CR. sirt2 regulates adipocyte differentiation through FoxO1 acetylation/deacetylation. Cell Metabolism. 2007;**6**:105-114. DOI: 10.1016/j.cmet.2007.07.003

[15] Picard F, Kurtev M, Chung N, Topark-Ngarm A, Senawong T, Machado De Oliveira R, et al. Sirt1 promotes fat mobilization in white adipocytes by repressing PPAR-gamma. Nature. 2004;**429**:771-776. DOI: 10.1038/nature02583

[16] Puri N, Sodhi K, Haarstad M, Kim DH, Bohinc S, Foglio E, et al. Heme induced oxidative stress attenuates sirtuin1 and enhances adipogenesis in mesenchymal stem cells and mouse preadipocytes. Journal of Cellular Biochemistry. 2012;**113**:1926-1935. DOI: 10.1002/jcb.24061

[17] Zhou Y, Zhou Z, Zhang W, Hu X, Wei H, Peng J, et al. sirt1 inhibits adipogenesis and promotes myogenic differentiation in C3H10T1/2 pluripotent cells by regulating Wnt signaling. Cell & Bioscience. 2015;**5**:61. DOI: 10.1186/s13578-015-0055-5

[18] Ahn J, Lee H, Jung CH, Jeon TI, Ha TY. MicroRNA-146b promotes adipogenesis by suppressing the sirt1-FOXO1 cascade. EMBO Molecular Medicine. 2013;**5**:1602-1612. DOI: 10.1002/emmm.201302647

[19] Wang F, Tong Q. sirt2 suppresses adipocyte differentiation by deacetylating FOXO1 and enhancing FOXO1's repressive interaction with PPARgamma. Molecular Biology of the Cell. 2009;**20**:801-808. DOI: 10.1091/mbc.E08-06-0647

[20] Wu YT, Chi KT, Lan YW, Chan JC, Ma YS, Wei YH. Depletion of Sirt3 leads to the impairment of adipogenic differentiation and insulin resistance via interfering mitochondrial function of adipose-derived human mesenchymal stem cells. Free Radical Research. 2018; **52**:1398-1415. DOI: 10.1080/10715762.2018.1489130

[21] Hong J, Li S, Wang X, Mei C, Zan L. Study of expression analysis of *sirt4* and the coordinate regulation of bovine adipocyte differentiation by *sirt4* and its transcription factors. Bioscience Reports. 2018;**38**(6):pii: BSR20181705. DOI: 10.1042/BSR20181705

[22] Chen Q, Hao W, Xiao C, Wang R, Xu X, Lu H, et al. sirt6 is essential for adipocyte differentiation by regulating mitotic clonal expansion. Cell Reports. 2017;**18**:3155-3166. DOI: 10.1016/j.celrep.2017.03.006

[23] Shin J, He M, Liu Y, Paredes S, Villanova L, Brown K, et al. sirt7 represses Myc activity to suppress ER stress and prevent fatty liver disease. Cell Reports. 2013;**5**:654-665. DOI: 10.1016/j.celrep.2013.10.007

[24] Fang J, Ianni A, Smolka C, Vakhrusheva O, Nolte H, Krüger M, et al. Sirt7 promotes adipogenesis in the mouse by inhibiting autocatalytic activation of Sirt1. Proceedings of the National Academy of Sciences of the United States of America. 2017;**114**: E8352-E8361. DOI: 10.1073/pnas.1706945114

[25] Qiang L, Wang L, Kon N, Zhao W, Lee S, Zhang Y, et al. Brown remodeling of white adipose tissue by SirT1-dependent deacetylation of Pparγ. Cell. 2012;**150**:620-632. DOI: 10.1016/j.cell.2012.06.027

[26] Abdesselem H, Madani A, Hani A, Al-Noubi M, Goswami N, Ben Hamidane H, et al. sirt1 limits adipocyte hyperplasia through c-Myc inhibition. The Journal of Biological Chemistry. 2016;**291**:2119-2135. DOI: 10.1074/jbc.M115.675645

[27] Shi T, Wang F, Stieren E, Tong Q. sirt3, a mitochondrial sirtuin deacetylase, regulates mitochondrial function and thermogenesis in brown adipocytes. The Journal of Biological Chemistry. 2005;**280**:13560-13567. DOI: 10.1074/jbc.M414670200

[28] Jin L, Galonek H, Israelian K, Choy W, Morrison M, Xia Y, et al. Biochemical characterization,

localization, and tissue distribution of the longer form of mouse sirt3. Protein Science. 2009;**18**:514-525. DOI: 10.1002/pro.50

[29] Lombard DB, Alt FW, Cheng HL, Bunkenborg J, Streeper RS, Mostoslavsky R, et al. Mammalian Sir2 homolog sirt3 regulates global mitochondrial lysine acetylation. Molecular and Cellular Biology. 2007;**27**:8807-8814. DOI: 10.1128/MCB.01636-07

[30] Shuai L, Zhang LN, Li BH, Tang CL, Wu LY, Li J, et al. sirt5 regulates brown adipocyte differentiation and browning of subcutaneous white adipose tissue. Diabetes. 2019;**68**(7):1449-1461. DOI: 10.2337/db18-1103

[31] Yao L, Cui X, Chen Q, Yang X, Fang F, Zhang J, et al. Cold-inducible sirt6 regulates thermogenesis of brown and beige fat. Cell Reports. 2017;**20**:641-654. DOI: 10.1016/j.celrep.2017.06.069

[32] Bordone L, Cohen D, Robinson A, Motta MC, van Veen E, Czopik A, et al. sirt1 transgenic mice show phenotypes resembling calorie restriction. Aging Cell. 2007;**6**:759-767. DOI: 10.1111/j.1474-9726.2007.00335.x

[33] Banks AS, Kon N, Knight C, Matsumoto M, Gutiérrez-Juárez R, Rossetti L, et al. SirT1 gain of function increases energy efficiency and prevents diabetes in mice. Cell Metabolism. 2008;**8**:333-341. DOI: 10.1016/j.cmet.2008.08.014

[34] Ye X, Li M, Hou T, Gao T, Zhu WG, Yang Y. Sirtuins in glucose and lipid metabolism. Oncotarget. 2017;**8**:1845-1859. DOI: 10.18632/oncotarget.12157

[35] Wang GL, Fu YC, Xu WC, Feng YQ, Fang SR, Zhou XH. Resveratrol inhibits the expression of SREBP1 in cell model of steatosis via Sirt1-FOXO1 signaling pathway. Biochemical and Biophysical Research Communications. 2009;**380**:644-649. DOI: 10.1016/j.bbrc.2009.01.163

[36] Hou X, Xu S, Maitland-Toolan KA, Sato K, Jiang B, Ido Y, et al. sirt1 regulates hepatocyte lipid metabolism through activating AMP-activated protein kinase. The Journal of Biological Chemistry. 2008;**283**:20015-20026. DOI: 10.1074/jbc.M802187200

[37] Li X, Zhang S, Blander G, Tse JG, Krieger M, Guarente L. sirt1 deacetylates and positively regulates the nuclear receptor LXR. Molecular Cell. 2007;**28**:91-106. DOI: 10.1016/j.molcel.2007.07.032

[38] Groen AK, Oude Elferink R, Verkade HJ, Kuipers F. The ins and outs of reverse cholesterol transport. Annals of Medicine. 2004;**36**:135-145

[39] Lin R, Tao R, Gao X, Li T, Zhou X, Guan KL, et al. Acetylation stabilizes ATP-citrate lyase to promote lipid biosynthesis and tumor growth. Molecular Cell. 2013;**51**:506-518. DOI: 10.1016/j.molcel.2013.07.002

[40] Hirschey MD, Shimazu T, Goetzman E, Jing E, Schwer B, Lombard DB, et al. sirt3 regulates mitochondrial fatty-acid oxidation by reversible enzyme deacetylation. Nature. 2010;**464**:121-125. DOI: 10.1038/nature08778

[41] Savastano S, Di Somma C, Colao A, Barrea L, Orio F, Finelli C, et al. Preliminary data on the relationship between circulating levels of Sirtuin 4, anthropometric and metabolic parameters in obese subjects according to growth hormone/insulin-like growth factor-1 status. Growth Hormone & IGF Research. 2015;**25**:28-33. DOI: 10.1016/j.ghir.2014.10.006

[42] Park J, Chen Y, Tishkoff DX, Peng C, Tan M, Dai L, et al. sirt5-mediated lysine desuccinylation impacts diverse metabolic pathways. Molecular

Cell. 2013;**50**:919-930. DOI: 10.1016/j.molcel.2013.06.001

[43] Nasrin N, Wu X, Fortier E, Feng Y, Bare' OC, Chen S, et al. sirt4 regulates fatty acid oxidation and mitochondrial gene expression in liver and muscle cells. The Journal of Biological Chemistry. 2010;**285**:31995-32002. DOI: 10.1074/jbc.M110.124164

[44] Kuang J, Zhang Y, Liu Q, Shen J, Pu S, Cheng S, et al. Fat-specific Sirt6 ablation sensitizes mice to high-fat diet-induced obesity and insulin resistance by inhibiting lipolysis. Diabetes. 2017; **66**:1159-1171. DOI: 10.2337/db16-1225

[45] Kanfi Y, Peshti V, Gil R, Naiman S, Nahum L, Levin E, et al. sirt6 protects against pathological damage caused by diet-induced obesity. Aging Cell. 2010; **9**:162-173. DOI: 10.1111/j.1474-9726.2009.00544.x

[46] Cioffi M, Vallespinos-Serrano M, Trabulo SM, Fernandez-Marcos PJ, Firment AN, Vazquez BN, et al. MiR-93 controls adiposity via inhibition of Sirt7 and Tbx3. Cell Reports. 2015;**12**: 1594-1605. DOI: 10.1016/j.celrep.2015.08.006

[47] Yoshizawa T, Karim MF, Sato Y, Senokuchi T, Miyata K, Fukuda T, et al. sirt7 controls hepatic lipid metabolism by regulating the ubiquitin-proteasome pathway. Cell Metabolism. 2014;**19**: 712-721. DOI: 10.1016/j.cmet.2014.03.006

[48] Yoshizaki T, Milne JC, Imamura T, Schenk S, Sonoda N, Babendure JL, et al. sirt1 exerts anti-inflammatory effects and improves insulin sensitivity in adipocytes. Molecular and Cellular Biology. 2009;**29**:1363-1374. DOI: 10.1128/MCB.00705-08

[49] Yoshizaki T, Schenk S, Imamura T, Babendure JL, Sonoda N, Bae EJ, et al. sirt1 inhibits inflammatory pathways in macrophages and modulates insulin sensitivity. American Journal of Physiology. Endocrinology and Metabolism. 2010;**298**:E419-E428. DOI: 10.1152/ajpendo.00417.2009

[50] Kauppinen A, Suuronen T, Ojala J, Kaarniranta K, Salminen A. Antagonistic crosstalk between NF-κB and sirt1 in the regulation of inflammation and metabolic disorders. Cellular Signalling. 2013;**25**:1939-1948. DOI: 10.1016/j.cellsig.2013.06.007

[51] Lappas M. Anti-inflammatory properties of sirtuin 6 in human umbilical vein endothelial cells. Mediators of Inflammation. 2012;**2012**: 597514. DOI: 10.1155/2012/597514

[52] Xiao C, Wang RH, Lahusen TJ, Park O, Bertola A, Maruyama T, et al. Progression of chronic liver inflammation and fibrosis driven by activation of c-JUN signaling in Sirt6 mutant mice. The Journal of Biological Chemistry. 2012;**287**:41903-41913. DOI: 10.1074/jbc.M112.415182

[53] Hui X, Zhang M, Gu P, Li K, Gao Y, Wu D, et al. Adipocyte sirt1 controls systemic insulin sensitivity by modulating macrophages in adipose tissue. EMBO Reports. 2017;**18**:645-657. DOI: 10.15252/embr.201643184

[54] Qiao L, Shao J. sirt1 regulates adiponectin gene expression through Foxo1-C/enhancer-binding protein alpha transcriptional complex. The Journal of Biological Chemistry. 2006; **281**:39915-39924. DOI: 10.1074/jbc.M607215200

[55] Zhang YY, Zhou LM. Omentin-1, a new adipokine, promotes apoptosis through regulating Sirt1-dependent p53 deacetylation in hepatocellular carcinoma cells. European Journal of Pharmacology. 2013;**698**:137-144. DOI: 10.1016/j.ejphar.2012

[56] Patel L, Buckels AC, Kinghorn IJ, Murdock PR, Holbrook JD, Plumpton C,

et al. Resistin is expressed in human macrophages and directly regulated by PPAR gamma activators. Biochemical and Biophysical Research Communications. 2003;**300**:472-476

[57] Carter S, Miard S, Roy-Bellavance C, Boivin L, Li Z, Pibarot P, et al. Sirt1 inhibits resistin expression in aortic stenosis. PLoS One. 2012;7:e35110. DOI: 10.1371/journal.pone.0035110

[58] Asadi S, Goodarzi MT, Saidijam M, Karimi J, Azari RY, Farimani AR, et al. Resveratrol attenuates visfatin and vaspin genes expression in adipose tissue of rats with type 2 diabetes. Iranian Journal of Basic Medical Sciences. 2015;**18**:537-543

[59] Howitz KT, Bitterman KJ, Cohen HY, Lamming DW, Lavu S, Wood JG, et al. Small molecule activators of sirtuins extend Saccharomyces cerevisiae lifespan. Nature. 2003;**425**:191-196. DOI: 10.1038/nature01960

[60] Rayalam S, Yang JY, Ambati S, Della-Fera MA, Baile CA. Resveratrol induces apoptosis and inhibits adipogenesis in 3T3-L1 adipocytes. Phytotherapy Research. 2008;**22**:1367-1371. DOI: 10.1002/ptr.2503

[61] Pearson KJ, Baur JA, Lewis KN, Peshkin L, Price NL, Labinskyy N, et al. Resveratrol delays age-related deterioration and mimics transcriptional aspects of dietary restriction without extending life span. Cell Metabolism. 2008;**8**:157-168. DOI: 10.1016/j.cmet.2008.06.011

[62] Timmers S, Konings E, Bilet L, Houtkooper RH, van de Weijer T, Goossens GH, et al. Calorie restriction-like effects of 30 days of resveratrol supplementation on energy metabolism and metabolic profile in obese humans. Cell Metabolism. 2011;**14**:612-622. DOI: 10.1016/j.cmet.2011.10.002

[63] Smith JJ, Kenney RD, Gagne DJ, Frushour BP, Ladd W, Galonek HL, et al. Small molecule activators of sirt1 replicate signaling pathways triggered by calorie restriction in vivo. BMC Systems Biology. 2009;**3**:31. DOI: 10.1186/1752-0509-3-31

[64] Mellini P, Valente S, Mai A. Sirtuin modulators: An updated patent review (2012–2014). Expert Opinion on Therapeutic Patents. 2015;**25**:5-15. DOI: 10.1517/13543776.2014.982532

[65] Milne JC, Lambert PD, Schenk S, Carney DP, Smith JJ, Gagne DJ, et al. Small molecule activators of sirt1 as therapeutics for the treatment of type 2 diabetes. Nature. 2007;**450**:712-716. DOI: 10.1038/nature06261

[66] Feige JN, Lagouge M, Canto C, Strehle A, Houten SM, Milne JC, et al. Specific sirt1 activation mimics low energy levels and protects against diet-induced metabolic disorders by enhancing fat oxidation. Cell Metabolism. 2008;**8**:347-538. DOI: 10.1016/j.cmet.2008.08.017

[67] Yamazaki Y, Usui I, Kanatani Y, Matsuya Y, Tsuneyama K, Fujisaka S, et al. Treatment with SRT1720, a sirt1 activator, ameliorates fatty liver with reduced expression of lipogenic enzymes in MSG mice. American Journal of Physiology. Endocrinology and Metabolism. 2009;**297**:E1179-E1186. DOI: 10.1152/ajpendo.90997.2008

[68] Pacholec M, Bleasdale JE, Chrunyk B, Cunningham D, Flynn D, Garofalo RS, et al. SRT1720, SRT2183, SRT1460, and resveratrol are not direct activators of sirt1. The Journal of Biological Chemistry. 2010;**285**:8340-8351. DOI: 10.1074/jbc.M109.088682

[69] Cantó C, Gerhart-Hines Z, Feige JN, Lagouge M, Noriega L, Milne JC, et al. AMPK regulates energy expenditure by modulating NAD+ metabolism and sirt1

activity. Nature. 2009;**458**:1056-1060. DOI: 10.1038/nature07813

[70] Dai H, Sinclair DA, Ellis JL, Steegborn C. Sirtuin activators and inhibitors: Promises, achievements, and challenges. Pharmacology & Therapeutics. 2018;**188**:140-154. DOI: 10.1016/j.pharmthera.2018.03.004

[71] Villalba JM, Alcaín FJ. Sirtuin activators and inhibitors. BioFactors. 2012;**38**:349-359. DOI: 10.1002/biof.1032

[72] Kuryłowicz A, Wicik Z, Owczarz M, Jonas MI, Kotlarek M, Świerniak M, et al. NGS reveals molecular pathways affected by obesity and weight loss-related changes in miRNA levels in adipose tissue. International Journal of Molecular Sciences. 2017;**19**:E66. DOI: 10.3390/ijms19010066

Chapter 3

Novel Aspects of Follistatin/ Transforming Growth Factor-β (TGF-β) Signaling in Adipose Tissue Metabolism: Implications in Metabolic Health

Shehla Pervin, Wilson Nyah, Srinivasa T. Reddy and Rajan Singh

Abstract

Obesity is a major risk factor for several metabolic disorders including insulin resistance, diabetes, and cardiovascular diseases. Chronic imbalance of calorie intake and expenditure results in storage of excess unused energy resulting in obesity and related metabolic dysfunctions. While most obesity therapies are focused on reducing the calorie intake and exercise, recent studies suggest that targeting cellular energy expenditure could be a fascinating alternative approach. Brown adipose tissue (BAT) not only has a remarkable calorie burning capacity, but it could also promote triglyceride clearance and glucose disposal. Induction of brown adipose mass and activity in relevant tissues are linked to relieve symptoms of various metabolic disorders such as diabetes, insulin resistance, and cardiovascular diseases. Follistatin (Fst), an extracellular protein that binds and antagonizes several members of the transforming growth factor beta (TGF-β)/myostatin (Mst) superfamily, promotes brown adipose characteristics in both white and brown adipose tissues by targeting distinct molecular pathways. Inhibition of Mst, on the other hand, leads to significant upregulation of adipose browning in white adipose tissues. This chapter will summarize most recent developments in targeting adipose tissue and their functional characteristics to explore therapeutic potential of Fst and TGF-β/Mst signaling to modulate adipose tissue metabolic functions to combat obesity and related metabolic syndromes.

Keywords: adipocyte, follistatin, myostatin, transforming growth factor beta, adipose browning, uncoupling protein 1, thermogenesis, insulin sensitivity

1. Introduction

Obesity is a global health problem that results from chronic imbalance between energy intake and its expenditure. Obesity is a major risk factor for several metabolic diseases including diabetes, dyslipidemia, insulin resistance, cardiovascular diseases, nonalcoholic fatty liver, and even some form of cancer. According to most recent global estimates, by year 2030 roughly 2.16 billion individuals will be obese as defined by body mass index (BMI) of 30 or higher [1]. The economic impact of obesity and related metabolic complications has been estimated between 4 and 8% of gross domestic product which is comparable to 2018 defense budget ($643 billion) and Medicare ($588 billion) in the United States [2]. Thus the toll of obesity imposes massive and rapidly growing economic cost beyond human suffering. This economic burden of obesity, therefore, significantly impacts low-income and otherwise disadvantaged population. Staying physically active and maintaining a healthy diet are well accepted and proven strategies to prevent weight gain; however, an alarming increase of global obesity urgently requires the development of novel and highly effective anti-obesity therapies. According to the laws of thermodynamics, any treatment for obesity must require reduced energy intake, increased energy expenditure, or both. Recent data suggest that targeting cellular bioenergetics may provide attractive therapeutic avenues for the treatment and prevention of obesity. White adipose tissue (WAT) and brown adipose tissue (BAT) are two distinct adipose tissue types present in mammals. While WAT with larger unilocular lipid droplets store excess energy in the form of triglycerides, BAT consisting of multilocular smaller lipid droplets enriched with mitochondria that express uncoupling protein 1 (UCP1) has specialized capacity to dissipate excess energy via activating non-shivering thermogenesis. Pockets of UCP1-positive adipocytes have also been found within WAT depots which are called beige or brite (brown within white) adipocytes. These beige adipocytes show some morphological and functional similarities to classical brown adipocytes present with the BAT. Several molecular signaling pathways are reported to play significant roles in the development and differentiation of these white, beige, and brown adipose cells. Transforming growth factor beta (TGF-β) controls the development, growth, and cellular functions of diverse cell types by transmitting signals via dual serine/threonine kinase receptors and transcription factors called Smads, especially Smad3. TGF-β expression levels are significantly elevated in adipose tissues from obese mice [3], and blocking of TGF-β/Smad3 signaling results in protection from obesity and diabetes. These metabolic benefits are associated with increased appearance of brown-like adipocytes within the WAT [4]. Inactivation of myostatin (Mst) also called growth and differentiation factor 8 (GDF8), a key member of the TGF-β superfamily in both differentiating mouse embryonic fibroblast (MEF) primary cultures from wild type (WT) and Mst knockout (Mst KO) embryos, as well as in white adipose tissues of Mst KO mouse models, displays beige adipocyte phenotype and upregulation of key beige markers compared to the wild type [5]. Blockade of activin receptor IIB (ActRIIB) that integrates the actions of Mst and TGF-β-related ligands has been demonstrated to activate functional brown adipogenesis and thermogenesis [6]. Inhibition of Smad3 signaling, which has been identified as canonical pathway for Mst, induced WAT browning [7]. It therefore suggests that antagonizing TGF-β/Smad3/Mst signaling pathway would lead to significant favorable metabolic alterations by promoting adipose browning. Since follistatin (Fst) is a well-known inhibitor of TGF-β signaling pathway in a variety of cell lines [8–10], and a key antagonist of Mst, Braga et al. [11] hypothesized that Fst may promote browning of white adipocytes, and using differentiating MEF primary cultures from WT and Fst KO embryos provided the first evidence that Fst is a novel inducer of brown adipose characteristics. Subsequent studies using Fst-transgenic (Fst-Tg) mice overexpressing Fst under the control of skeletal muscle-specific myosin light chain promoter, the authors demonstrated that Fst targets distinct pathways to promote brown adipose characteristics in both BAT and WAT [11]. Combined together, these findings support the idea that targeting TGF-β/Smad3/Mst signaling either via direct genetic or pharmacological inhibition of this pathways or via directly upregulating Fst could be attractive therapeutic options for the treatment of obesity and related metabolic diseases.

2. Developmental origin, transcriptional regulators, and molecular signature of beige and brown adipocytes

Although white and brown adipocytes share many common features such as PPAR-γ-driven transcriptional control of adipogenesis, their gene expression profiles are distinct, and they do not share a direct common progenitor. Recent genetic studies using fat-mapping experiments have shown that while brown fat in the interscapular region and skeletal muscle share some common features and are derived from Myf5 expressing (Myf5+) cells (previously assumed to be exclusively present in committed skeletal muscle precursors), these Myf5+ precursor cells were absent in white and beige cells [12, 13]. Studies from several other laboratories using global gene expression as well as mitochondrial proteomics signature confirmed that BAT is highly related to the skeletal muscle and not WAT [14, 15]. The divergence of brown adipocyte precursor and skeletal muscle was investigated using Pax7, another myogenic marker in pulse-chase experiments, and it was reported that this divergence occurred between embryonic day 9.5 and 11.5 in mice [16]. UCP1-expressing beige adipocytes present in epididymal WAT (Epi WAT) are thought to be derived through the proliferation and differentiation of platelet-derived growth factor receptor α (PDGRF α), CD44, and SC1 precursor cells [17]. Beige or brown-like cells in the inguinal WAT, on the other hand, are suggested to be derived from Myf5-negative (Myf5-) precursor cells [12]. However, this view has recently been challenged by various groups on the basis of linage analysis studies that suggest that subsets of white adipocytes are derived from both Myf5+ and Myf5- precursors and respond to beta-3 adrenergic receptor (β3-AR) signaling suggesting that these beige adipocytes may have multiple origins [18–20]. A subset of UCP1-positive beige adipocytes is also recently reported to arise from Myh11, selectively expressed in smooth muscle cells [21]. It is also possible that beige cells can either originate from mesodermal stem cells or trans-differentiation of mature white adipocytes [22]. Beige cells may also originate from Ebf2+ precursors located in the subcutaneous adipose tissue (SAT) population characterized by specific markers Cd137 and Tmeme26 [23]. Furthermore, it is also possible that thermogenic adipocytes may arise from endothelial cells and capillaries where retinoic acid (RA) could induce adipose browning by activating VEGF signaling pathways [24]. RA is known to trigger angiogenesis and facilitate de novo generation of *Pdgrfα* expressing adipocyte precursors mediated via VEGFA/VEGFR2 signaling [25]. These findings, therefore, collectively suggest that beige adipocytes which are composed of heterogeneous cell populations may have distinct cellular origins.

The acquisition of morphological and molecular features of brown and beige fat is under the control of PPARγ-coactivator 1α (PGC-1α) [26]. PGC-1α is induced early in brown fat differentiation and is preferentially expressed in mature brown adipocytes. PGC1-1α ectopic expression is sufficient to promote various aspects of differentiation toward the brown fat lineage. PGC-1α is also rapidly and highly induced by cold exposure and turns on several key components of the adaptive thermogenic program including fatty acid oxidation, mitochondrial biogenesis, and increased oxygen consumption [27]. The expression levels of 140kD zinc figure containing transcription factor called PR domain containing 16 (PRDM16) are very high in BAT compared to the visceral WAT and appear to play a major role in brown adipose/skeletal muscle fate determination [28]. Ectopic expression of PRDM16 in cultured mesenchymal cells including white preadipocytes induced a complete brown fat differentiation program and activation of key thermogenic (*Ucp1*, *Pgc-1α*, *cidea*, and *elov3*) genes and coactivates the transcriptional activity of PGC-1α/PGC-1β, as well as PPARα and PPARγ [12, 28]. Coincident with these changes, PRDM16 expression also led to suppression of several white fat and muscle-selective markers [29]. On the other hand, genetic ablation of PRDM16 in brown fat leads to significant increase in white adipose and muscle-specific genes [28]. These findings, therefore, suggest that PRDM16 acts as a critical cell fate regulator of brown fat, and careful analysis of its embryonic expression pattern will be extremely valuable to dissect out the putative brown fat-skeletal muscle precursors. Signaling molecules that control the timing and specificity of PRDM16 expression during development are unknown. Certain growth factors like bone morphogenetic proteins (BMPs), members of the TGF-β superfamily of secreted factors, are reported to influence both brown and white adipocyte differentiation [30–32]. While BMP2 and BMP4 are reported to promote white adipose cell differentiation, BMP7 is reported to selectively induce brown adipogenesis in committed precursor cells [32, 33]. BMP7 exposure to fibroblast cultures results in induction of full brown fat differentiation program, including induction of PRDM16 and UCP1 expression [30]. Importantly, significantly reduced amounts of BAT mass were observed in BMP7-deficient mice. However, it is not clear whether BMP7 plays any role in the regulation of PRDM16.

Under basal conditions both beige and brown adipocytes share some of the same key markers including UCP1 and PRDM16; however, data from clonal cell lines suggest that beige and brown adipose cells express related but distinctly different gene expression profiles [23]. Beige cells are highly enriched in Tmem26, Tbx1, and CD137 expression [23]. Comprehensive gene expression analysis of adipose tissues isolated from interscapular BAT and inguinal fat revealed several other beige-selective genes including *Ear2*, *Sp100*, *Klh113*, and *Slc27a* [23]. Molecular profiling and histological analysis of human BAT identified additional beige-selective markers HoxC8, HoxC9, Cited1, and Shox2 [34, 35]. On the other hand, classical brown adipocytes selectively express epithelial V-like antigen (Eva 1), Zic1, Lhx1, and Epsti [23, 36–38]. Using adipose tissues isolated from white and interscapular BAT from 129SVE mice, Wu et al. identified additional genes including *Hspb7*, *Ebf3*, *Pdk4*, *Fbxo31*, and *Oplah* that were enriched in BAT [23]. Using a combination of in silico, in vitro, as well as in vivo approaches, Ussar et al. reported the identification of three new cell surface markers of adipose tissues [39]. In this study, amino acid transporter Asc1 was identified as a white adipocyte-specific cell surface protein with very low to undetectable levels in brown adipocytes, whereas amino acid transporter PAT2 and the purinergic receptor P2RX5 are cell surface markers expressed in classical brown and beige adipocytes.

Studies from microRNA (miRNA) signature analysis between beige and brown adipogenesis have provided significant differences in their molecular signature. MiRNA-193b-365 cluster is expressed in brown fat tissues and initially thought to be involved in the regulation of brown fat differentiation by inhibiting Runx1t1, which inhibits BAT differentiation [40]. However, subsequent in vivo studies show a normal BAT function in the absence of miRNA-193b-365 [41]. Inhibition of miRNA-182 and miRNA-203 in brown adipocytes led to downregulation of several genes involved in oxidative phosphorylation and electron transport [42]. Inhibition of miRNA-106b-93 led to induced expression of several adipogenic markers [43]. Similarly, positive (miRNA-196b) and negative (miRNA-26) regulation of beige adipogenesis have been identified [44, 45]. miRNAs that positively (miRNA-30 family) and negatively (miRNA-27 and miRNA-34a) regulate both brown and beige adipocytes are also identified [46–48]. Thus, there appear to be clear differences between BAT and beige miRNA gene signature in mouse and human tissues and cells.

3. Role of transforming growth factor-β (TGF-β) superfamily in adipose browning and metabolic health

The TGF-β superfamily consists of more than 33 members including TGFβ1, TGFβ2, and TGFβ3, bone morphogenetic proteins (BMPs), growth differentiation factors (GDFs), and activins that play important roles in growth, development, and function of diverse cell types including adipocytes [49, 50]. These evolutionary highly conserved superfamily members transmit their signals via dual serine/threonine kinase receptors and transcription factors called Smads. TGF-β superfamily members control various aspects of adipocyte biology. Adipose tissues from obese mice were reported to express elevated levels of TGF-β [3]. The binding of TGF-β family to their membrane receptors could be somewhat promiscuous and may allow 7 type I and 5 type II receptors to transduce signaling from these TGF-β superfamily members. Multiple cell types including adipose progenitors, preadipocytes, and adipocytes along with various immune cells are known to express protein belonging to TGF-β superfamily and their antagonists [51]. The role of TGF-β/Smad3 signaling in regulating beige adipocyte phenotype and metabolic characteristics were elegantly demonstrated by Yadav et al. [4]. They observed significant positive correlation between TGF-β1 levels and adiposity in both rodents and human subjects. Using Smad3$^{-/-}$ mice, they provided interesting link between Smad3 loss and protection against diet-induced obesity and related metabolic syndromes. These changes in metabolic parameters were associated with induction of white to brown phenotype and significantly increased mitochondrial biogenesis. In the same study, examination of a total of 184 nondiabetic human subjects from diverse ethnic groups, the authors identified direct relationship between circulating TGF-β1 levels and BMI, fat mass, and VO_2 consumption. Furthermore, anti-TGF-β antibody in Lep$^{ob/ob}$ and diet-induced obesity mouse models resulted in significantly reduced body weight, improved glucose and insulin tolerance, as well as significantly reduced fasting glucose and insulin levels. These metabolic improvements were associated with elevated expression of BAT/mitochondria-specific proteins in white adipose tissues. Such links between TGF-β signaling and mitochondrial energy metabolism pathway have also been reported by several other laboratories [52, 53]. Extracellular matrix protein microfibril-associated glycoprotein (MAGP) was found to be significantly altered in obese humans, and inactivation of MAGP1 gene (Mfap2$^{-/-}$) resulted in adipocyte hypertrophy and predisposition to metabolic diseases. Mfap2$^{-/-}$ mice had significantly lower expression of UCP1 expression in BAT and display reduced subcutaneous adipose browning and defective adaptation to cold exposure [53]. Treatment of these Mfap2$^{-/-}$ mice with neutralizing concentrations of anti-TGF-β antibody led to decreased adiposity and improved body temperature. Administration of a novel activin receptor type II B (ActRIIB) decoy receptor containing the extracellular domain of ActRIIB fused to human Fc (ActRIIB-Fc) resulted in suppression of diet-induced obesity and associated metabolic functions in mice [54]. In the same study, significantly increased adipose browning in epididymal white fat displaying robustly increased expression of UCP1 and PGC 1-α was observed following ActRIIB-Fc treatment. Furthermore, protection from diet-induced obesity in ActRIIB-Fc-treated mice was demonstrated to result from increased energy expenditure and not decreased caloric intake. Combined together, these interesting findings suggest novel insights into the role of TGF-β signaling in suppressing adipose browning program within white fat tissues in both mouse models and human subjects suggesting that efficient blockade of TGF-β activity could serve as an effective treatment strategy for obesity and diabetes.

Myostatin (Mst) is a key member of the TGF-β superfamily which is known to play a major role in the regulation of skeletal muscle growth. However, recent studies have clearly indicated that the effect of Mst extends beyond its role in skeletal muscle. Genetic deletion of Mst displays favorable changes in several metabolic parameters including decreased fat deposition, enhanced fatty acid oxidation, improved insulin sensitivity, and increased resistance to diet-induced obesity besides increased skeletal muscle mass [55, 56]. Since Mst is expressed at very low levels in adipose tissues [57], it remains unclear how depletion of Mst can suppress fat accumulation. Earlier studies by Kim et al. show that treatment of mouse primary brown preadipocytes with recombinant Mst led to significant inhibition of brown adipogenic differentiation and reduced expression of markers *Ucp1*, *Prdm16*, and *Pgc-1α* [58]. A comparison of key thermogenic markers obtained from epididymal (Epi) and subcutaneous (SC) white adipose tissues shows significantly increased expression of UCP1 and PRDM16 in Mst KO mice compared to the WT littermates [54]. Using differentiating primary cultures isolated from WT and Mst KO mouse embryonic fibroblasts (MEFs) in the same study, Braga et al. further confirmed upregulation of key thermogenic markers in Mst KO mice compared to the WT mice [5]. Furthermore, recombinant Mst protein treatment of the differentiating MEFs significantly downregulated several key thermogenic markers including UCP1, PRDM16, PGC-1α/PGC-1β, and BMP7. Also, protein expression of adiponectin and phosphorylated AMP-activated protein kinase (pAMPK), which control the expression of genes involved in energy metabolism in coordination with NAD+-dependent sirtuin 1 (SirT1), were upregulated in Mst KO MEFs compared to the WT group [59, 60]. In another study, Chio et al. reported significantly increased energy expenditure and leptin sensitivity in Mst-deficient mice that could explain low fat mass in these mice compared to the WT group [61]. Shan et al. demonstrated that inhibition of Mst signaling in WAT SVF cells failed to induce browning of white adipocytes in vitro, suggesting that loss or inhibition of Mst signaling in preadipocytes does not account for adipose browning in white adipocyte tissues in Mst KO mice [62]. In order to test the possible non-cell autonomous effects of Mst, the authors thoroughly analyzed various muscle-derived circulating factors that could account for the browning phenotype. They reported that skeletal muscle-derived Fndc5 (irisin) plays a central role in mediating white adipose browning in Mst KO mice via activation of AMPK-PGC1α-Fndc5 pathway, suggesting the involvement of muscle-adipose cross talk during the process [63, 64]. Fndc5/irisin was initially identified as a PGC-1α-dependent myokine that is responsible for adipose browning both in vitro and in vivo and protects diet-induced obesity in obesity [65]. Possible involvement of Fndc5 in mediating adipose browning in Mst loss-of-function models has emerged from other laboratories. Dong et al. also confirmed possible intermediate role for Fndc5/irisin-mediated adipose browning in Mst KO mice. In another study, Mst signaling was shown to regulate Fndc5 expression and adipose browning via upregulation of miRNA-34a. Several laboratories have demonstrated that the absence of Mst in both in vitro and in vivo models improves insulin sensitivity [58, 66]. Several other laboratories provided additional evidence to support the view that Mst loss-of-function results in significant metabolic improvements resulting from adipose browning. Increased insulin sensitivity and WAT browning were reported in Meishan pigs with Mst functional deletion [67]. Several browning-related genes including UCP1, PGC-1α, PRDM16, Cidea, CD137, and Tmem26 were significantly upregulated in these Mst-deficient pigs. Protein expression levels of insulin receptor (IR) and insulin receptor substrate (IRS) were significantly induced in the skeletal muscle of these Mst-deficient pigs. Interestingly, serum irisin levels and skeletal muscle protein expression of irisin precursor protein FNDC5 were significantly higher in Mst-null pigs than wild-type pigs. These authors also demonstrated that inhibition of irisin expression was unable to block the activation of insulin signaling pathway, thus, implying that irisin may not be required for activation of insulin signaling in Mst-deficient skeletal muscle [67]. Genetic disruption of Mst ($Mst^{-/-}$) in $LDLR^{-/-}$ ($Mst^{-/-}/LDLR^{-/-}$) mice was shown to reduce the development of proatherogenic dyslipidemia, improve insulin-mediated glucose disposal, and protect against hepatic steatosis [68]. Furthermore, Guo et al. demonstrated that administration of adeno-associated virus 9 (AAV9)-mediated Mst-pro-peptide in adult $LDLR^{-/-}$ mice reduced diet-induced hepatosteatosis and progression of atherosclerosis [69]. In both these reports, the beneficial metabolic effects were claimed to result from enlarged muscle mass following inactivation of functional Mst in $LDLR^{-/-}$ mice. Several recent reports have provided strong evidence suggesting that brown fat activation could reduce hypercholesterolemia and protect from atherosclerosis development [70–72]. Therefore, it is possible that observed beneficial effects of Mst inactivation in $LDLR^{-/-}$ background could be mediated at least in part via adipose browning.

More recently, Mst expression has been linked to mediate BAT-muscle cross talk [73]. Induction of Mst following loss of interferon regulatory factor 4 (IRF4) in BAT leads to significantly reduced exercise capacity, ribosomal protein synthesis, and mitochondrial function [73]. On the other hand, reduced serum levels of Mst resulting from IRF4 overexpression significantly increased exercise capacity in muscle. IRF4 expression was found to be induced in brown adipocytes following cold exposure and β3-adrenergic receptor (AR) agonist [74]. IRF4 expression was reported to be sufficient to induce thermogenic program in BAT, and loss of IRF4 in brown fat leads to significantly reduced energy expenditure. Also, IRF4 was shown to physically and functionally interact with PGC-1α to upregulate transcription of *Ucp1* gene and drive mitochondrial biogenesis and thermogenic program in BAT. In light of these exciting reports establishing IRF4 as a novel inhibitor of Mst, it is not surprising that IRF4 could antagonize the bioactivity of secreted Mst present in the blood to promote overall thermogenic program.

4. Follistatin regulation of white and brown adipose characteristics

Follistatin (Fst) is a soluble secreted glycoprotein that is known to bind and neutralize the activity of several members of the TGF-β superfamily including activins and Mst in a variety of cell lines [9–10, 77]. Several genetic studies have convincingly demonstrated an essential role of Fst in the regulation of muscle mass. Elegant initial studies led by Lee and McPherron demonstrated that inhibition of Mst either by genetic manipulation or overexpressing Fst resulted in significantly increased muscle mass in mice [75]. The direct role for Fst in the regulation of muscle mass was also verified by several laboratories [8, 9, 76]. Fst was identified as a downstream target of testosterone during its pro-myogenic action in both in vitro and in vivo studies [8, 9]. Testosterone treatment of mouse mesenchymal multipotent C3H 10T1/C3H 10T2 cells led to upregulation of Fst and altered the expression of several key members of TGF-β superfamily [8]. Testosterone-induced upregulation of key myogenic markers MyoD and myosin heavy chain II proteins in C3H 10T1/C3H 10 T2 cells was abolished in cells simultaneously treated with anti-Fst antibody, suggesting an essential role of Fst during testosterone regulation of myogenic differentiation. The essential role of Fst was also established in in vivo studies using castrated male mice, where Fst gene expression level significantly reduced in the levator ani (LA) muscle compared to the sham-operated male mice, but testosterone supplementation in castrated mice upregulated Fst mRNA expression in LA muscle to the baseline levels [8]. Subsequent studies by Braga et al. reported that primary culture of muscle satellite cells express Fst and respond to testosterone treatment. Fst blocked TGF-β-induced inhibition of MHC II expression and induction of Smad2/Smad3 phosphorylation in satellite cells [9]. These reports provide conclusive evidence that Fst plays an important role in promoting myogenic differentiation and increasing muscle mass. In spite of several reports demonstrating as essential role of Fst in regulating muscle mass and its function, its role in lipid metabolism and energy balance was largely unknown. Fst-deficient mice die within hours after birth and have several defects including reduced size of diaphragm muscle [76]. These severe musculoskeletal defects were suggested to account for the neonatal death of these Fst-deficient pups. Since maintenance of body temperature through thermogenesis during early hours of neonatal life is extremely important, and both skeletal muscle and thermogenic brown fat share Myf5+ precursor cells, it is logical to test whether Fst could play a role in regulating the thermogenic program along with its established role in muscle development. Based on this logic and several published reports that Fst can bind and antagonize the biological actions of TGF-β/Mst signaling [8, 9], which are known inhibitors of thermogenic program, Braga et al. hypothesized that Fst may promote adipose browning and favorably alter energy metabolism [11]. Initial quantitative analysis of Fst gene expression in a mouse tissue panel consisting of several metabolic tissues demonstrated that Fst expression was highest in BAT along with skeletal muscle and was also expressed at a substantial level in inguinal WAT and the liver [11]. The expression levels in other tissues including the heart, intestine, and testis were significantly lower. This finding for the first time suggested a possible novel role of Fst in BAT and WAT and led to a series of subsequent in vitro and in vivo experimental approaches to delineate the precise role of Fst in adipose tissues of both origins. Using immortalized mouse brown preadipocytes, the authors clearly demonstrated that Fst protein expression was significantly induced in differentiated BAT cells displaying characteristic multilocular lipid droplets compared to the undifferentiated cells [11]. As expected, levels of key brown adipose markers such as UCP1 and PRDM16 were also significantly induced after differentiation of BAT cells. Furthermore, Fst gene expression in BAT was dramatically induced following cold exposure of the mice, suggesting that Fst is a novel cold-inducible gene and could play important role in regulating key metabolic functions. Since Fst KO mice are not viable, Braga et al. utilized primary cultures of differentiating mouse embryonic fibroblast (MEF) cultures isolated from Fst KO and WT embryos to test whether Fst loss-of-function results in defective thermogenic program [11]. Significant impairment in adipogenic differentiation and upregulation of BAT-specific markers were noted in Fst-deficient MEF cultures compared to the WT. Exogenous recombinant Fst protein treatment was able to rescue the thermogenic genes and proteins in Fst-deficient MEF cultures and further induced the expression of several BAT-specific genes in differentiated mouse BAT cells. Affymetrix global gene expression profiling clearly demonstrated lipid metabolism as the most significantly altered pathway and identified several genes involved in lipid metabolism and energy production such as *Adn*, *Thrsp*, *Hp*, *Acsl1*, *Fabp4*, *Pparg*, and *Cd36* were significantly downregulated in Fst KO MEFs compared to the WT. Significantly lower basal mitochondrial respiration in Fst KO MEFs compared to the WT cultures was rescued by exogenous recombinant Fst, suggesting that Fst increases cellular respiration [11].

In subsequent experiments, Singh et al. explored the in vivo actions of Fst overexpression on both white and brown adipose tissues using Fst-transgenic (Fst-Tg) mice to determine whether Fst promotes adipose browning and brown adipose mass and function in these mice and identify possible molecular targets of Fst in these adipose tissues. Fst-Tg mice express Fst under a muscle-specific promoter [75] in which the circulating Fst levels are 1.5-fold higher along with ~70% increased interscapular BAT mass compared to the WT mice [77]. BAT signature genes and several key proteins involved in mitochondrial biogenesis, fatty acid oxidation (FAO), were significantly upregulated in iBAT as well as in Epi and SC adipose tissues of Fst-Tg mice compared to the WT mice [77]. The BAT marker UCP1 and beige-specific markers CD137 were significantly higher in both WAT depots of Fst-Tg mice compared to WT, with relatively larger differences observed in SC adipose depots. Several other markers involved in mitochondrial biogenesis and FAO were also found to be induced in both adipose depots from Fst-Tg mice compared to the WT mice. These observed differences in adipose browning capacity between the two WAT depots were found to be consistent with previous reports [78].

The actions of Fst in regulating WAT and BAT adipose characteristics were shown to be mediated via two distinct mechanisms. Fst increased phosphorylation of p38 mitogen-activated protein kinase (p38 MAPK) and extracellular signal-regulated kinase (ERK1/ERK2) in both WAT depots, while it increased Myf5 expression in iBAT of Fst-Tg mice [77]. The authors utilized in vitro studies to further confirm the obligatory and mechanistic basis for these distinctly different Fst targets. In differentiating 3T3-L1 cells, recombinant Fst treatment led to significant induction of UCP1 and beige-specific marker CD137. Pharmacological inhibition of p38 MAPK and ERK1/ERK2 phosphorylation by SB023580 (10 μM) and PD98059 (10 μM), respectively, either alone or in combination, led to significant blockade of Fst-induced (i) phosphorylation of both these proteins as expected and (ii) upregulation of UCP1 protein [77]. On the other hand, in BAT and differentiated mouse BAT cells, Fst increased Myf5 protein expression. Knockdown of Myf5 expression led to significant inhibition of recombinant Fst-mediated increase in UCP1 protein expression in differentiated mouse BAT cells. Additionally, Fst treatment was able to rescue Myf5 gene and protein expression in Fst KO MEFs, reinforcing that Myf5 is a critical mediator of Fst action in BAT [77]. Since BAT and skeletal muscle share Myf5-expressing progenitor cells [78, 79], the authors proposed that Fst promotes BAT activation and skeletal muscle growth by upregulating Myf5. Based on these novel findings, the authors proposed that Fst induces Myf5 expression in BAT and Myf5-positive progenitor cells to increase classical BAT activation, whereas it promotes phosphorylation of p38MAPK and ERK1/ERK2 in WAT to promote adipose browning. It is also possible that Fst could efficiently enhance the production of one or more of several myokines which are shown to induce white adipose browning including irisin (encoded by *Fndc5* gene), IL6, or FGF21 [80–82]. Both Fst and FGF21 were shown to be induced and secreted following exercise [81]. Also, secretion of irisin by skeletal muscle in response to exercise was reported to induce phosphorylation of p38 MAPK and ERK1/ERK2 leading to white adipose browning [80]. Upregulation of *Fndc5* gene expression was reported in skeletal muscle after treatment with both recombinant Fst protein and anti-Mst antibody [62], suggesting that Fst could target irisin/Mst-mediated pathway in muscle tissue to promote adipose browning mediated via muscle-adipose cross talk. Using similar MEF-based primary cultures obtained from WT and Fst KO and Mst KO, Braga et al. showed reciprocal regulation of BMP7 [5, 11], a key driver of brown adipogenesis and energy metabolism by Fst and Mst. These findings were confirmed by other laboratories in support of Fst-induced upregulation of BMP7 [83] and its downregulation by Mst [84]. Gene expression analysis of MEF primary cultures from WT and Fst KO versus WT and Mst KO shows several genes that were reciprocally regulated by Fst and Mst as identified by Affymetrix gene expression analysis and further validated by quantitative real-time PCR analysis (**Figure 1**). Analysis of basal oxygen consumption rate (OCR) in differentiated MEF cultures from these WT and Fst/Mst KO groups further suggests reciprocal effects of Fst and Mst on mitochondrial respiration (**Figure 2**). Combined together, these findings support the view that Fst may exert its pro-browning effects at least in part by inhibiting Mst signaling. Follistatin-like-3 (FSTL3) has been reported as another Mst binding protein that

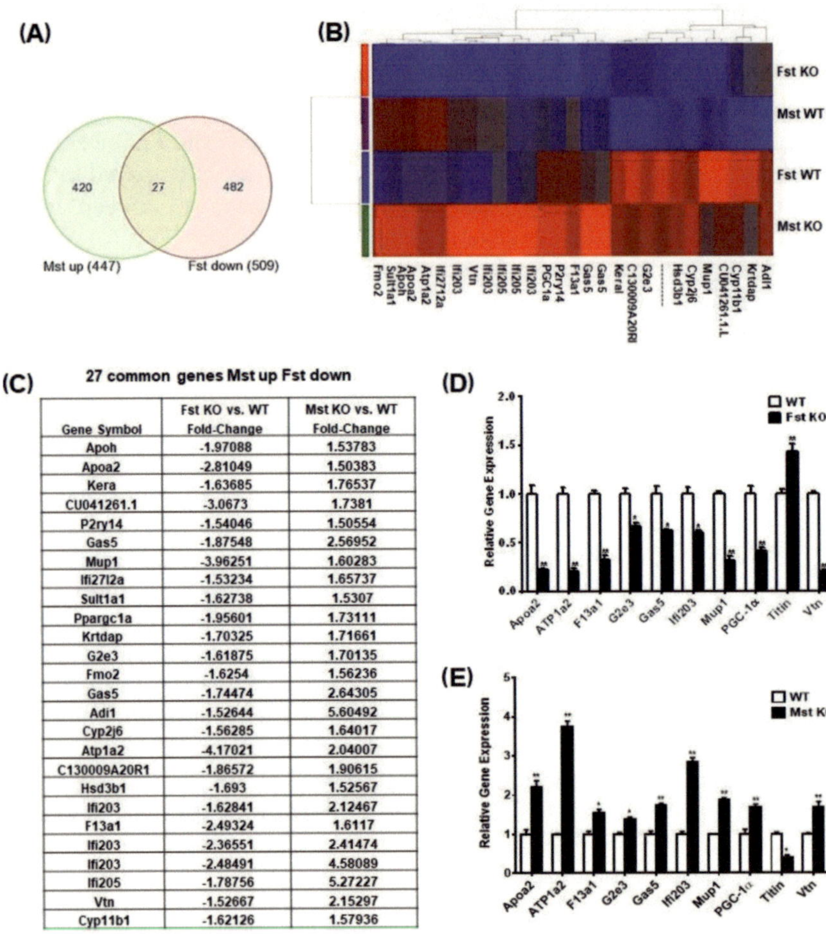

Gene Symbol	Fst KO vs. WT Fold-Change	Mst KO vs. WT Fold-Change
Apoh	-1.97088	1.53783
Apoa2	-2.81049	1.50383
Kera	-1.63685	1.76537
CU041261.1	-3.0673	1.7381
P2ry14	-1.54046	1.50554
Gas5	-1.87548	2.56952
Mup1	-3.96251	1.60283
Ifi27l2a	-1.53234	1.65737
Sult1a1	-1.62738	1.5307
Ppargc1a	-1.95601	1.73111
Krtdap	-1.70325	1.71661
G2e3	-1.61875	1.70135
Fmo2	-1.6254	1.56236
Gas5	-1.74474	2.64305
Adi1	-1.52644	5.60492
Cyp2j6	-1.56285	1.64017
Atp1a2	-4.17021	2.04007
C130009A20R1	-1.86572	1.90615
Hsd3b1	-1.693	1.52567
Ifi203	-1.62841	2.12467
F13a1	-2.49324	1.6117
Ifi203	-2.36551	2.41474
Ifi203	-2.48491	4.58089
Ifi205	-1.78756	5.27227
Vtn	-1.52667	2.15297
Cyp11b1	-1.62126	1.57936

Figure 1.
*Reciprocal effects of Fst and Mst on several genes involved in lipid and energy metabolism. Primary cultures obtained from differentiating WT and Fst/Mst KO cells were analyzed by Affymetrix global gene profiling. (A) Van diagram showing 27 common genes that were reciprocally regulated by Fst and Mst. (B) Heat map showing differential expression of those 27 genes. (C) List of reciprocally regulated common genes. (D, E) Validation of Affymetrix data real-time PCR analysis. n = 3; *p ≤ 0.05; **p ≤ 0.01.*

could play an important role in regulating fat mass and glucose homeostasis [85]. FSTL3 knockout mice display distinct phenotype including decreased fat mass and improved insulin sensitivity. However, it is not known whether FSTL3 regulates BAT mass and thermogenic activity, suggesting that the role of Fst may be more complicated [86].

Activation of p38MAPK pathway that promotes adipose browning by β3-adrenergic receptor (β3-AR) has been well documented [87, 88]. Since intraperitoneal injection of β3-AR agonist CL316,243 in Fst-Tg mice resulted in additive response to UCP1 levels in WAT and BAT compared to the WT mice, it is possible that β3-AR signaling could play an important role upstream of p38 MAPK pathway during Fst-induced adipose browning. More recently, elegant studies by Liu et al. demonstrated that inhibition of follicle-stimulating hormone (FSH) through a polyclonal antibody induced adipose browning and activated BAT and thermogenesis [89]. Since Fst was initially isolated from follicular fluid and found to inhibit secretion of FSH from anterior pituitary, this recent report further validates the identification of Fst as a novel inducer of adipose browning.

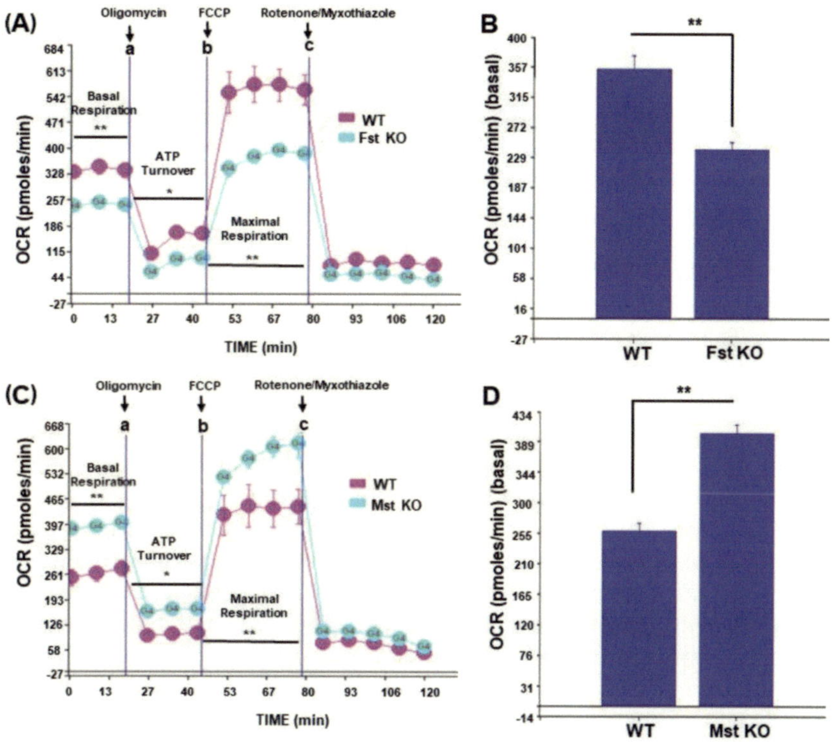

Figure 2.
Reciprocal effects of Fst (A, B) and Mst (C, D) on basal oxygen consumption rate (OCR) as analyzed by the seahorse bioscience XF24 extracellular flux analyzer. Data are expressed as mean +/− SEM. $^{*}p \leq 0.05$; $^{**}p \leq 0.01$.

5. Metabolic profiling of Fst overexpression and relevance to metabolic diseases

In order to get better understanding of observed adipose browning and its metabolic consequences in Fst overexpressing in mice (Fst-Tg) as well as in differentiated 3T3-L1 (3T3-L1 Fst) preadipocyte, Singh et al. initially performed quantitative analysis of abdominal fat volume by CT scan, glucose clearance, and serum lipid profiles [90]. Fst-Tg mice displayed significant decrease in abdominal fat mass, increased glucose clearance, and significantly lower triglyceride (TG) and free fatty acid (FFA) levels compared to the WT control mice. A comparison of the overall lipidomic profiles using gas chromatography time-of-flight technology (GC TOF) shows a general reduction in diglycerides (DG), triglycerides (TG), ceramide (D42:0), fatty acids (FA), phosphatidylcholine (PC), phosphatidylethanolamine (PE), and lysophosphatidylethanolamines (LPE: 16.0) in Fst overexpressing 3T3-L1 (3T3-L1 Fst) cells compared to the basal 3T3-L1 cells after adipogenic differentiation (ref). On the other hand, a significant increase in several lysophosphatidylcholines (LPC) including LPC 16:0, LPC 18:0, and LPC 18:1 was observed in 3T3-L1 Fst cells in comparison to 3T3-L1 cells. The decreased levels of several of these lipid metabolites observed in 3T3-L1 Fst cells are known contributors toward the development of obesity and related metabolic diseases [91, 92]. Increased levels of several of these LPCs following Fst overexpression also suggest a beneficial role for Fst as these LPCs are reported to be significantly reduced in obesity and type 2 diabetes [93, 94]. Comprehensive analysis of metabolites obtained from epi and SC adipose tissue between WT and Fst-Tg mice provided significant differences between metabolites involved in energy and lipid metabolism of the groups. Several components of the Krebs cycle including citrate, succinylcarnitine, and fumarate were significantly downregulated in Fst-Tg Epi tissues compared to the WT tissues, whereas only reduced levels of succinate were found in SC adipose tissues form Fst-Tg mice compared to the WT mice. Also, several long-chain FAs, components of the carnitine metabolism, glycerolipids, ketone bodies, and lysolipids were selectively found to be lower in Fst-Tg Epi tissues than the WT group. Interestingly, levels of Epi cholesterol levels were also selectively reduced in Epi tissues only. Several key amino acids including tyrosine, components of tryptophan, branched-chain amino acid (BCAA), and urea cycle metabolism were also found to be dramatically reduced in Epi adipose tissues in Fst-Tg mice compared to the WT mice. A comparison of omega-3 polyunsaturated fatty acid (ω-3 PUFAs) levels between the groups shows highly significant increase selectively in SC adipose tissues of Fst-Tg mice. Interestingly, ω-3 PUFAs are reported to improve not only obesity-associated metabolic disorders including insulin resistance and dyslipidemia but also several aspects of energy and lipid metabolism and inflammation [95–97]. Significantly decreased levels of beta-hydroxybutyric acid (BHBA), the end product of FA beta-oxidation and key contributor to metabolic syndrome, were also observed in the Epi adipose tissues of Fst-Tg mice compared to the WT. Combined together, these comprehensive metabolomic profilings of Fst in vitro and in vivo overexpression show a clear pattern of favorable changes in several metabolites implicated in metabolic complications and provide future impetus to thoroughly investigate the novel therapeutic role of Fst.

6. Conclusions

Several lines of evidence support the view that brown and beige adipocytes play important roles in regulating various aspects of lipid and glucose metabolism. The browning process in WAT that entails a shift in WAT primary function from storing excess energy to the dissipation of energy has been linked to the prevention of progression and development of obesity and related metabolic abnormalities including insulin resistance, hyperlipidemia, and type 2 diabetes. Data generated from several laboratories collectively suggest that blocking of TGF-β/Smad3/Mst signaling efficiently increases brown adipose phenotypic and metabolic characteristics and possible downstream mediators during the process as summarized in **Figure 3**.

Accordingly, new strategies to identify and develop novel TGF-β/Mst inhibitors to increase BAT and beige adipose mass and activities are currently being explored with the hope that blockade of this signaling pathway could lead to the development of therapeutic avenues. Since Fst has been demonstrated to efficiently antagonize Mst and inhibit overall TGF-β signaling in several in vitro and in vivo models, the novel therapeutic potential of Fst for the treatment of obesity and related metabolic diseases needs to be thoroughly explored in preclinical studies. It is, therefore, necessary to identify the key molecular and cellular targets of Fst responsible for its regulation of overall thermogenic program. Although phosphorylation and activation of the p38MAPK/ERK1/ERK2 signaling by Fst in WAT have recently been linked to Fst-induced browning, the possible intermediate role of irisin during the process could not be ruled out. Similar to Fst, secretion of irisin by skeletal muscle is induced following exercise which could induce p38MAPK/ERK1/ERK2 phosphorylation and lead to browning of WAT [80]. Fibroblast growth factor 21 (FGF21), another exercise-induced secretory protein linked to adipose browning and which promotes brown adipose characteristics, has also been shown to be influenced by recombinant Fst (rFst) treatment in 3T3-L1 as well as in WAT of

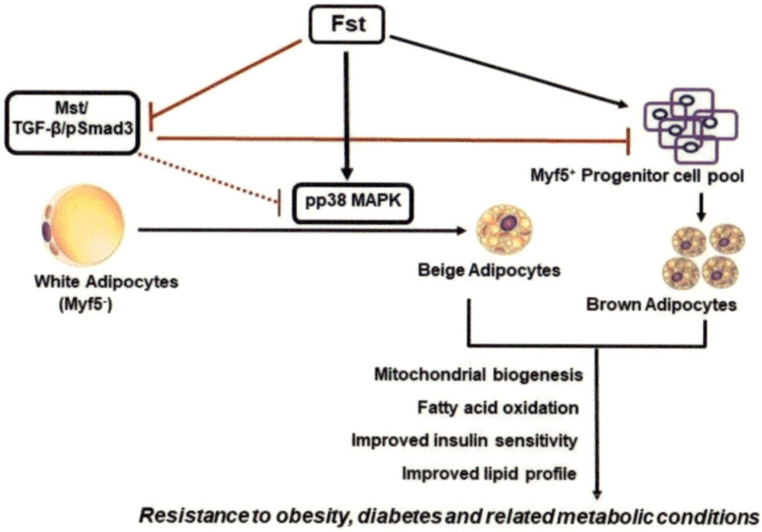

Figure 3.
Proposed hypothetical model for Fst and Mst/TGF-β regulation of adipose browning characteristics of white and brown adipose tissue and their metabolic implications.

Fst-transgenic (Fst-Tg) mice. Robust upregulation of FGF21/adiponectin/AMPK signaling pathway observed under both conditions suggests a possible mechanistic link between Fst and FGF21. Preclinical studies using an alternatively spliced cDNA of follistatin (FS344) delivered by adeno-associated virus (AAV) to muscle in both human patients with certain degenerative muscle disorders [98, 99] and nonhuman primates [100] show no apparent structural or functional aberrations in a variety of organs, suggesting the potential of Fst use in clinical trials, although these studies did not assess adipose tissue metabolic parameters. Therefore, novel antagonists of TGF-β/Mst signaling pathways, including Fst [101], hold a great promise for the treatment of not only muscle loss and dysfunction but also for obesity and related metabolic diseases.

Acknowledgements

This work was supported by the National Institute of Health Grants SC1AG049682 (RS), SC1CA1658650 (SP), UHI grant S21MD000103 and Accelerating Excellence in Translational Science (AXIS) U54MD007598 to Charles R. Drew University of Medicine and Science.

Author details

Shehla Pervin[1,2], Wilson Nyah[3], Srinivasa T. Reddy[1,4] and Rajan Singh[1,2]*

1 Department of Obstetrics and Gynecology, David Geffen School of Medicine at UCLA, Los Angeles, CA, USA

2 Division of Endocrinology and Metabolism, Charles R. Drew University of Medicine and Science, Los Angeles, CA, USA

3 College of Science and Health, Charles R. Drew University of Medicine and Science, Los Angeles, CA, USA

4 Department of Molecular and Medical Pharmacology, David Geffen School of Medicine at UCLA, Los Angeles, CA, USA

*Address all correspondence to: rajansingh@mednet.ucla.edu

References

[1] Tam CS, Lecoultre V, Ravussin E. Brown adipose tissue: Mechanisms and potential therapeutic targets. Circulation. 2012;**125**:2782-2791

[2] The Toll of America's Obesity. The New York Times. Available from: https://www.nytimes.com/2018/08/09/opinion/cost-diabetes-obesity-budget.html

[3] Samad F, Yamamoto K, Pandey M, Loskutoff DJ. Elevated expression of transforming growth factor-beta in adipose tissue from obese mice. Molecular Medicine. 1997;**3**:37-48

[4] Yadav H, Quijano C, Kamaraju AK, Gavrilova O, Malek R, Chen W, et al. Protection from obesity and diabetes by blockade of TGF-β/Smad3 signaling. Cell Metabolism. 2011;**14**:67-79

[5] Braga M, Pervin S, Norris K, Bhasin S, Singh R. Inhibition of in vitro and in vivo brown fat differentiation program by myostatin. Obesity. 2013;**21**:1180-1188

[6] Fournier B, Murray B, Gutzwiller S, Marcaletti S, Marcellin D, Bergling S, et al. Blockade of the activin receptor IIb activates functional brown adipogenesis and thermogenesis by inducing mitochondrial oxidative metabolism. Molecular and Cellular Biology. 2012;**32**:2871-2879

[7] Tiano JP, Springer DA, Rane SG. SMAD3 negatively regulates serum irisin and skeletal muscle FNDC5 and peroxisome proliferator-activated receptor γ coactivator 1-α (PGC-1α) during exercise. The Journal of Biological Chemistry. 2015;**290**:7671-7684

[8] Singh R, Bhasin S, Braga M, Artaza JN, Pervin S, Taylor WE, et al. Regulation of myogenic differentiation by androgens: Cross talk between androgen receptor/beta-catenin and follistatin/transforming growth factor-beta signaling pathways. Endocrinology. 2009;**150**:1259-1268

[9] Braga M, Bhasin S, Jasuja R, Pervin S, Singh R. Testosterone inhibits transforming growth factor-β signaling during myogenic differentiation and proliferation of mouse satellite cells: Potential role of follistatin in mediating testosterone action. Molecular and Cellular Endocrinology. 2012;**350**:39-52

[10] Pervin S, Singh V, Tucker A, Collazo J, Singh R. Modulation of transforming growth factor-β/follistatin signaling and white adipose browning: Therapeutic implications for obesity related disorders. Hormone Molecular Biology and Clinical Investigation. 2017;**31**(2)

[11] Braga M, Reddy ST, Vergnes L, Pervin S, Grijalva V, Stout D, et al. Follistatin promotes adipocyte differentiation, browning, and energy metabolism. Journal of Lipid Research. 2014;**55**:375-384

[12] Seale P, Bjork B, Yang W, Kajimura S, Chin S, Kuang S, et al. PRDM16 controls a brown fat/skeletal muscle switch. Nature. 2008;**454**:961-967

[13] Kajimura S, Seale P, Spiegelman BM. Transcriptional control of brown fat development. Cell Metabolism. 2010;**11**:257-262

[14] Timmons JA, Wennmalm K, Larsson O, Walden TB, Lassmann T, Petrovic N, et al. Myogenic gene expression signature establishes that brown and white adipocytes originate from distinct cell lineages. Proceedings of the National Academy of Sciences of the United States of America. 2007;**104**:4401-4406

[15] Forner F, Kumar C, Luber CA, Fromme T, Klingenspor M, Mann M.

Proteome differences between brown and white fat mitochondria reveal specialized metabolic functions. Cell Metabolism. 2009;**10**:324-335

[16] Lepper C, Fan CM. Inducible lineage tracing of Pax7-descendant cells reveals embryonic origin of adult satellite cells. Genesis. 2010;**48**:424-436

[17] Wang W, Seale P. Control of brown and beige fat development. Nature Reviews Molecular Cell Biology. 2016;**17**:691-702

[18] Sanchez-Gurmaches J, Hung CM, Sparks CA, Tang Y, Li H, Guertin DA. PTEN loss in the Myf5 lineage redistributes body fat and reveals subsets of white adipocytes that arise from Myf5 precursors. Cell Metabolism. 2012;**16**:348-362

[19] Lee YK, Cowan CA. White to brite adipocyte transition and back again. Nature Cell Biology. 2013;**15**:568-569

[20] Rosenwald M, Perdikari A, Rülicke T, Wolfrum C. Bi-directional interconversion of brite and white adipocytes. Nature Cell Biology. 2013;**15**:659-667

[21] Long JZ, Svensson KJ, Tsai L, Zeng X, Roh HC, Kong X, et al. A smooth muscle-like origin for beige adipocytes. Cell Metabolism. 2014;**19**:810-820

[22] Harms M, Seale P. Brown and beige fat: Development, function and therapeutic potential. Nature Medicine. 2013;**19**:1252-1263

[23] Wu J, Boström P, Sparks LM, Ye L, Choi JH, Giang AH, et al. Beige adipocytes are a distinct type of thermogenic fat cell in mouse and human. Cell. 2012;**150**:366-376

[24] Gupta RK, Mepani RJ, Kleiner S, Lo JC, Khandekar MJ, Cohen P, et al. Zfp423 expression identifies committed preadipocytes and localizes to adipose endothelial and perivascular cells. Cell Metabolism. 2012;**15**:230-239

[25] Wang B, Fu X, Liang X, Deavila JM, Wang Z, Zhao L, et al. Retinoic acid induces white adipose tissue browning by increasing adipose vascularity and inducing beige adipogenesis of PDGFRα+ adipose progenitors. Cell Discovery. 2017;**3**:17036

[26] Puigserver P, Wu Z, Park CW, Graves R, Wright M, Spiegelman BM. A cold-inducible coactivator of nuclear receptors linked to adaptive thermogenesis. Cell. 1998;**92**:829-839

[27] Wu Z, Puigserver P, Andersson U, Zhang C, Adelmant G, Mootha V, et al. Mechanisms controlling mitochondrial biogenesis and respiration through the thermogenic coactivator PGC-1. Cell. 1999;**98**:115-124

[28] Seale P, Kajimura S, Yang W, Chin S, Rohas LM, Uldry M, et al. Transcriptional control of brown fat determination by PRDM16. Cell Metabolism. 2007;**6**:38-54

[29] Kajimura S, Seale P, Tomaru T, Erdjument-Bromage H, Cooper MP, Ruas JL, et al. Regulation of the brown and white fat gene programs through a PRDM16/CtBP transcriptional complex. Genes & Development. 2008;**22**:1397-1409

[30] Tseng YH, Kokkotou E, Schulz TJ, Huang TL, Winnay JN, Taniguchi CM, et al. New role of bone morphogenetic protein 7 in brown adipogenesis and energy expenditure. Nature. 2008;**454**:1000-1004

[31] Nishimura R, Hata K, Ikeda F, Matsubara T, Yamashita K, Ichida F, et al. The role of Smads in BMP signaling. Frontiers in Bioscience. 2003;**8**:s275-s284

[32] Blázquez-Medela AM, Jumabay M, Boström KI. Beyond the bone: Bone

morphogenetic protein signaling in adipose tissue. Obesity Reviews. 2019;**20**:648-658

[33] Jin W, Takagi T, Kanesashi SN, Kurahashi T, Nomura T, Harada J, et al. Schnurri-2 controls BMP-dependent adipogenesis via interaction with Smad proteins. Developmental Cell. 2006;**10**:461-471

[34] Wang W, Kissig M, Rajakumari S, Huang L, Lim HW, Won KJ, et al. Ebf2 is a selective marker of brown and beige adipogenic precursor cells. Proceedings of the National Academy of Sciences of the United States of America. 2014;**111**:14466-14471

[35] Lidell ME, Betz MJ, Dahlqvist Leinhard O, Heglind M, Elander L, Slawik M, et al. Evidence for two types of brown adipose tissue in humans. Nature Medicine. 2013;**19**:631-634

[36] Sharp LZ, Shinoda K, Ohno H, Scheel DW, Tomoda E, Ruiz L, et al. Human BAT possesses molecular signatures that resemble beige/brite cells. PLoS One. 2012;7:e49452

[37] Petrovic N, Walden TB, Shabalina IG, Timmons JA, Cannon B, Nedergaard J. Chronic peroxisome proliferator-activated receptor gamma (PPARgamma) activation of epididymally derived white adipocyte cultures reveals a population of thermogenically competent, UCP1-containing adipocytes molecularly distinct from classic brown adipocytes. The Journal of Biological Chemistry. 2010;**285**:7153-7164

[38] Jespersen NZ, Larsen TJ, Peijs L, Daugaard S, Homøe P, Loft A, et al. A classical brown adipose tissue mRNA signature partly overlaps with brite in the supraclavicular region of adult humans. Cell Metabolism. 2013;**17**:798-805

[39] Ussar S, Lee KY, Dankel SN, Boucher J, Haering MF, Kleinridders A, et al. ASC-1, PAT2, and P2RX5 are cell surface markers for white, beige, and brown adipocytes. Science Translational Medicine. 2014;**6**:247ra103

[40] Sun L, Xie H, Mori MA, Alexander R, Yuan B, Hattangadi SM, et al. Mir193b-365 is essential for brown fat differentiation. Nature Cell Biology. 2011;**13**:958-965

[41] Feuermann Y, Kang K, Gavrilova O, Haetscher N, Jang SJ, Yoo KH, et al. MiR-193b and miR-365-1 are not required for the development and function of brown fat in the mouse. RNA Biology. 2013;**10**(12):1807-1814

[42] Kim HJ, Cho H, Alexander R, Patterson HC, Gu M, Lo KA, et al. MicroRNAs are required for the feature maintenance and differentiation of brown adipocytes. Diabetes. 2014;**63**:4045-4056

[43] Wu Y, Zuo J, Zhang Y, Xie Y, Hu F, Chen L, et al. Identification of miR-106b-93 as a negative regulator of brown adipocyte differentiation. Biochemical and Biophysical Research Communications. 2013;**438**:575-580

[44] Mori M, Nakagami H, Rodriguez-Araujo G, Nimura K, Kaneda Y. Essential role for miR-196a in brown adipogenesis of white fat progenitor cells. PLoS Biology. 2012;**10**:e1001314

[45] Liu W, Bi P, Shan T, Yang X, Yin H, Wang YX, et al. miR-133a regulates adipocyte browning in vivo. PLoS Genetics. 2013;**9**:e1003626

[46] Hu F, Wang M, Xiao T, Yin B, He L, Meng W, et al. miR-30 promotes thermogenesis and the development of beige fat by targeting RIP140. Diabetes. 2015;**64**:2056-2068

[47] Sun L, Trajkovski M. MiR-27 orchestrates the transcriptional regulation of brown adipogenesis. Metabolism. 2014;**63**:272-282

[48] Fu T, Seok S, Choi S, Huang Z, Suino-Powell K, Xu HE, et al. MicroRNA 34a inhibits beige and brown fat formation in obesity in part by suppressing adipocyte fibroblast growth factor 21 signaling and SIRT1 function. Molecular and Cellular Biology. 2014;**34**:4130-4142

[49] Budi EH, Duan D, Derynck R. Transforming growth factor-β receptors and Smads: Regulatory complexity and functional versatility. Trends in Cell Biology. 2017;**27**:658-672

[50] Shi Y, Massagué J. Mechanisms of TGF-beta signaling from cell membrane to the nucleus. Cell. 2003;**113**:685-700

[51] Lee MJ. Transforming growth factor beta superfamily regulation of adipose tissue biology in obesity. Biochimica et Biophysica Acta—Molecular Basis of Disease. 1864;**2018**:1160-1171

[52] Casalena G, Daehn I, Bottinger E. Transforming growth factor-β, bioenergetics, and mitochondria in renal disease. Seminars in Nephrology. 2012;**32**:295-303

[53] Craft CS, Pietka TA, Schappe T, Coleman T, Combs MD, Klein S, et al. The extracellular matrix protein MAGP1 supports thermogenesis and protects against obesity and diabetes through regulation of TGF-β. Diabetes. 2014;**63**(6):1920-1932

[54] Koncarevic A, Kajimura S, Cornwall-Brady M, Andreucci A, Pullen A, Sako D, et al. A novel therapeutic approach to treating obesity through modulation of TGFβ signaling. Endocrinology. 2012;**153**:3133-3146

[55] Lebrasseur NK. Building muscle, browning fat and preventing obesity by inhibiting myostatin. Diabetologia. 2012;**55**:13-17

[56] Bernardo BL, Wachtmann TS, Cosgrove PG, Kuhn M, Opsahl AC, Judkins KM, et al. Postnatal PPARdelta activation and myostatin inhibition exert distinct yet complimentary effects on the metabolic profile of obese insulin-resistant mice. PLoS One. 2010;**5**:e11307

[57] Feldman BJ, Streeper RS, Farese RV Jr, Yamamoto KR. Myostatin modulates adipogenesis to generate adipocytes with favorable metabolic effects. Proceedings of the National Academy of Sciences of the United States of America. 2006;**103**:15675-15680

[58] Kim WK, Choi HR, Park SG, Ko Y, Bae KH, Lee SC. Myostatin inhibits brown adipocyte differentiation via regulation of Smad3-mediated β-catenin stabilization. The International Journal of Biochemistry & Cell Biology. 2012;**44**(2):327-334

[59] Scherer PE, Williams S, Fogliano M, Baldini G, Lodish HF. A novel serum protein similar to C1q, produced exclusively in adipocytes. The Journal of Biological Chemistry. 1995;**270**:26746-26749

[60] Hu E, Liang P, Spiegelman BM. AdipoQ is a novel adipose-specific gene dysregulated in obesity. The Journal of Biological Chemistry. 1996;**271**:10697-10703

[61] Choi SJ, Yablonka-Reuveni Z, Kaiyala KJ, Ogimoto K, Schwartz MW, Wisse BE. Increased energy expenditure and leptin sensitivity account for low fat mass in myostatin-deficient mice. American Journal of Physiology. Endocrinology and Metabolism. 2011;**300**:E1031-E1037

[62] Shan T, Liang X, Bi P, Kuang S. Myostatin knockout drives browning of white adipose tissue through activating the AMPK-PGC1α-Fndc5 pathway in muscle. The FASEB Journal. 2013;**27**:1981-1989

[63] Rodríguez A, Becerril S, Ezquerro S, Méndez-Giménez L, Frühbeck G.

Crosstalk between adipokines and myokines in fat browning. Acta Physiologica. 2017;**219**(2):362-381

[64] Stanford KI, Goodyear LJ. Muscle-adipose tissue cross talk. Cold Spring Harbor Perspectives in Medicine. 2018;**8**(8):pii: a029801

[65] Boström P, Wu J, Jedrychowski MP, Korde A, Ye L, Lo JC, et al. A PGC1-α-dependent myokine that drives brown-fat-like development of white fat and thermogenesis. Nature. 2012;**481**(7382):463-468

[66] Ge X, Sathiakumar D, Lua BJ, Kukreti H, Lee M, McFarlane C. Myostatin signals through miR-34a to regulate Fndc5 expression and browning of white adipocytes. International Journal of Obesity. 2017;**41**(1):137-148

[67] Cai C, Qian L, Jiang S, Sun Y, Wang Q, Ma D, et al. Loss-of-function myostatin mutation increases insulin sensitivity and browning of white fat in Meishan pigs. Oncotarget. 2017;**8**(21):34911-34922

[68] Tu P, Bhasin S, Hruz PW, Herbst KL, Castellani LW, Hua N, et al. Genetic disruption of myostatin reduces the development of proatherogenic dyslipidemia and atherogenic lesions in Ldlr null mice. Diabetes. 2009;**58**(8):1739-1748

[69] Guo W, Wong S, Bhasin S. AAV-mediated administration of myostatin pro-peptide mutant in adult Ldlr null mice reduces diet-induced hepatosteatosis and arteriosclerosis. PLoS One. 2013;**8**(8):e71017

[70] Berbée JF, Boon MR, Khedoe PP, Bartelt A, Schlein C, Worthmann A, et al. Brown fat activation reduces hypercholesterolaemia and protects from atherosclerosis development. Nature Communications. 2015;**6**:6356

[71] Bartelt A, John C, Schaltenberg N, Berbée JFP, Worthmann A, Cherradi ML, et al. Thermogenic adipocytes promote HDL turnover and reverse cholesterol transport. Nature Communications. 2017;**8**:15010

[72] Hoeke G, Kooijman S, Boon MR, Rensen PC, Berbée JF. Role of brown fat in lipoprotein metabolism and atherosclerosis. Circulation Research. 2016;**118**:173-182

[73] Kong X, Yao T, Zhou P, Kazak L, Tenen D, Lyubetskaya A, et al. Brown adipose tissue controls skeletal muscle function via the secretion of myostatin. Cell Metabolism. 2018;**28**:631-643

[74] Kong X, Banks A, Liu T, Kazak L, Rao RR, Cohen P, et al. IRF4 is a key thermogenic transcriptional partner of PGC-1α. Cell. 2014;**158**:69-83

[75] Lee SJ, McPherron AC. Regulation of myostatin activity and muscle growth. Proceedings of the National Academy of Sciences of the United States of America. 2001;**98**:9306-9311

[76] Matzuk MM, Lu N, Vogel H, Sellheyer K, Roop DR, Bradley A. Multiple defects and perinatal death in mice deficient in follistatin. Nature. 1995;**374**:360-363

[77] Singh R, Braga M, Reddy ST, Lee SJ, Parveen M, Grijalva V, et al. Follistatin targets distinct pathways to promote brown adipocyte characteristics in brown and white adipose tissues. Endocrinology. 2017;**158**:1217-1230

[78] Lo KA, Sun L. Turning WAT into BAT: A review on regulators controlling the browning of white adipocytes. Bioscience Reports. 2013;**33**(5):pii: e00065

[79] Sanchez-Gurmaches J, Guertin DA. Adipocyte lineages: Tracing back the origins of fat. Biochimica et Biophysica Acta. 1842;**2014**:340-351

[80] Zhang Y, Li R, Meng Y, Li S, Donelan W, Zhao Y, et al. Irisin

stimulates browning of white adipocytes through mitogen-activated protein kinase p38 MAP kinase and ERK MAP kinase signaling. Diabetes. 2014;**63**:514-525

[81] Hansen JS, Pedersen BK, Xu G, Lehmann R, Weigert C, Plomgaard P. Exercise-induced secretion of FGF21 and follistatin are blocked by pancreatic clamp and impaired in type 2 diabetes. The Journal of Clinical Endocrinology and Metabolism. 2016;**101**:2816-2825

[82] Reza MM, Subramaniyam N, Sim CM, Ge X, Sathiakumar D, McFarlane C, et al. Irisin is a pro-myogenic factor that induces skeletal muscle hypertrophy and rescues denervation-induced atrophy. Nature Communications. 2017;**8**:1104

[83] Amthor H, Christ B, Rashid-Doubell F, Kemp CF, Lang E, Patel K. Follistatin regulates bone morphogenetic protein-7 (BMP-7) activity to stimulate embryonic muscle growth. Developmental Biology. 2002;**243**:115-127

[84] Rebbapragada A, Benchabane H, Wrana JL, Celeste AJ, Attisano L. Myostatin signals through a transforming growth factor beta-like signaling pathway to block adipogenesis. Molecular and Cellular Biology. 2003;**23**:7230-7242

[85] Brown ML, Bonomi L, Ungerleider N, Zina J, Kimura F, Mukherjee A, et al. Follistatin and follistatin like-3 differentially regulate adiposity and glucose homeostasis. Obesity. 2011;**19**:1940-1949

[86] Mukherjee A, Sidis Y, Mahan A, Raher MJ, Xia Y, Rosen ED, et al. FSTL3 deletion reveals roles for TGF-beta family ligands in glucose and fat homeostasis in adults. Proceedings of the National Academy of Sciences of the United States of America. 2007;**104**(4):1348-1353

[87] Collins S, Surwit RS. The beta-adrenergic receptors and the control of adipose tissue metabolism and thermogenesis. Recent Progress in Hormone Research. 2001;**56**:309-328

[88] Cao W, Medvedev AV, Daniel KW, Collins S. Beta-adrenergic activation of p38 MAP kinase in adipocytes: cAMP induction of the uncoupling protein 1 (UCP1) gene requires p38 MAP kinase. The Journal of Biological Chemistry. 2001;**276**:27077-27082

[89] Liu P, Ji Y, Yuen T, Rendina-Ruedy E, DeMambro VE, Dhawan S, et al. Blocking FSH induces thermogenic adipose tissue and reduces body fat. Nature. 2017;**546**:107-112

[90] Singh R, Pervin S, Lee SJ, Kuo A, Grijalva V, David J, et al. Metabolic profiling of follistatin overexpression: A novel therapeutic strategy for metabolic diseases. Diabetes, Metabolic Syndrome and Obesity: Targets and Therapy. 2018;**11**:65-84

[91] Xia JY, Holland WL, Kusminski CM, Sun K, Sharma AX, Pearson MJ, et al. Targeted induction of ceramide degradation leads to improved systemic metabolism and reduced hepatic steatosis. Cell Metabolism. 2015;**22**:266-278

[92] Chimin P, Andrade ML, Belchior T, Paschoal VA, Magdalon J, Yamashita AS, et al. Adipocyte mTORC1 deficiency promotes adipose tissue inflammation and NLRP3 inflammasome activation via oxidative stress and de novo ceramide synthesis. Journal of Lipid Research. 2017;**58**:1797-1807

[93] Barber MN, Risis S, Yang C, Meikle PJ, Staples M, Febbraio MA, et al. Plasma lysophosphatidylcholine levels are reduced in obesity and type 2 diabetes. PLoS One. 2012;**7**:e41456

[94] Kim JY, Park JY, Kim OY, Ham BM, Kim HJ, Kwon DY, et al. Metabolic

profiling of plasma in overweight/obese and lean men using ultra performance liquid chromatography and Q-TOF mass spectrometry (UPLC-Q-TOF MS). Journal of Proteome Research. 2010;**9**:4368-4375

[95] Martínez-Fernández L, Laiglesia LM, Huerta AE, Martínez JA, Moreno-Aliaga MJ. Omega-3 fatty acids and adipose tissue function in obesity and metabolic syndrome. Prostaglandins & Other Lipid Mediators. 2015;**121** (Pt A):24-41

[96] Kunesová M, Braunerová R, Hlavatý P, Tvrzická E, Stanková B, Skrha J, et al. The influence of n-3 polyunsaturated fatty acids and very low calorie diet during a short-term weight reducing regimen on weight loss and serum fatty acid composition in severely obese women. Physiological Research. 2006;**55**:63-72

[97] Krebs JD, Browning LM, McLean NK, Rothwell JL, Mishra GD, Moore CS, et al. Additive benefits of long-chain n-3 polyunsaturated fatty acids and weight-loss in the management of cardiovascular disease risk in overweight hyperinsulinaemic women. International Journal of Obesity. 2006;**30**:1535-1544

[98] Mendell JR, Sahenk Z, Al-Zaidy S, Rodino-Klapac LR, Lowes LP, Alfano LN, et al. Follistatin gene therapy for sporadic inclusion body myositis improves functional outcomes. Molecular Therapy. 2017;**25**:870-879

[99] Mendell JR, Sahenk Z, Malik V, Gomez AM, Flanigan KM, Lowes LP, et al. A phase 1/2a follistatin gene therapy trial for Becker muscular dystrophy. Molecular Therapy. 2015;**23**:192-201

[100] Kota J, Handy CR, Haidet AM, Montgomery CL, Eagle A, Rodino-Klapac LR, et al. Follistatin gene delivery enhances muscle growth and strength in nonhuman primates. Science Translational Medicine. 2009;**1**:6ra15

[101] Singh R. Composition and methods for treating or preventing metabolic syndrome disorders. US 9,682,093 B2 patent; 2017. Available from: https://patentimages.storage.googleapis.com/67/27/b3/e5ee5a9cd485d9/US9682093.pdf

Chapter 4

Effect of Alcohol on Gut-Liver Axis and Adipose Tissue

Dhara Patel and Palash Mandal

Abstract

Adipose tissue comprises of large volumes of biologically functioning fat globule, which employs substantial systemic effect. Adipocytes and adipokines play an active role in autocrine, paracrine, or endocrine metabolic functions. Recent studies demonstrated that the hormonal role of adipocyte and adipose tissue dysfunction contributes to the pathogenesis of alcoholic liver disease (ALD) by the activation of CYP2E1. The gut microbiome and adipose tissue response play a pivotal role in the pathogenesis of ALD. Enteric dysbiosis increases plasma levels of metabolites that activate Kupffer cells. Recent literature suggested that chronic alcohol consumption is also correlated with oxidative stress in adipose tissue, inflammation, and adipocyte cell death, decrease in adiponectin, increase level of leptin and resistin, adipose tissue mass, and insulin resistance that acts on the muscle and liver. Dysbiosis combined with non-nutritional diet has an effect on the luminal metabolism causing immunological changes in the gut that might also contribute to pathogenesis of nonalcoholic fatty liver disease (NAFLD). Understanding the interaction between the altered gut microbiota, diet, environmental factors, and their effects on the gut-liver axis can provide an insight toward the pathogenesis of liver-associated disease.

Keywords: alcoholic liver disease, adipose tissue, adipokines, gut microbiota, nonalcoholic fatty liver disease

1. Introduction

Alcohol is considered the fifth leading risk factor for premature death and various disorders universally. It is psychoactive substance that leads to overuse of alcohol or alcoholism abuse. Alcohol related liver diseases are the primary cause of every third person undergoing liver transplants worldwide. Worldwide, alcohol liver disease (ALD) causes 14.5 million disability-reduced life years and approximately 500,000 deaths in 2010 [1]. Depending on behavior, genetics, and comorbidities, individuals who consume alcohol develop hepatic steatosis, an early stage of alcoholic hepatitis [2]. Although ALD is a disease that requires an intention for consumption of alcohol, there are various other factors, including genetic host system characteristics involved in the development and progression. The amount of pure alcohol consumption and duration is directly linked to cirrhosis.

Adipose tissue comprises of large volumes of biologically functioning fat globule, which employs considered to be submissive [3]. Researchers have established a remarkable understanding of adipocytes being an acute component of metabolic pathways and functioning of endocrine organs. Recent studies have given an insight on the hormonal role of adipocytes. Adipose tissue is identified to secrete proteins that are termed as adipokines, which play an active role in autocrine, paracrine, or endocrine metabolic functions. Adiponectin, leptin, and resistin are the most affected functional adipokines.

The body as a whole is affected on the consumption of alcohol. It has been demonstrated that mainly enteric dysbiosis plays a significant role in the development of ALD. Due to an increased intestinal gut permeability of microbes like *Clostridiales*, *Ruminococcaceae*, and *Bifidobacterium* spp., this leads to an elevated plasma levels of metabolites like lipopolysaccharide (LPS), Toll like receptors (TLR-4, TLR-2), cell surface receptor and differentiation marker 14 (CD-14), NADPH oxidase homolog 4 (Nox-4), glucose transporter-4 (GLUT4), and short-chain fatty acid (SCFA) which activates Kupffer cells along with the consequent effects of inflammation, necrosis, and oxidative stress. The activation of cytochrome P450 2E1 (CYP2E1) mediated by ethanol breakdown leads to adipokine dysfunction. Adiponectin acts as an anti-inflammatory cytokine while leptin and resistin act as pro-inflammatory cytokines that trigger adenosine monophosphate-activated protein kinase (AMPK) pathway which activates fatty acid oxidation and decreased hepatic lipid influx and de novo lipogenesis. Studies have reported that chronic alcohol consumption leads to reduce levels of adiponectin and an increase in leptin secretion and macrophage migration inhibitory factor (MIF) leading to reduction in adipose tissue mass and increase in fatty acid uptake by hepatocytes [3, 4]. Compounds like rosiglitazone, a PPAR-Υ agonist that targets the adipocytes exogenously, have shown to attenuate alcohol-induced fatty liver [5, 6]. Inflammation due to bacterial translocation is the main contributor to the development of alcoholic liver disease. Cytokines like tumor necrosis factor alpha (TNF-α), interleukins (IL-1β, IL6, IL8), induced nitric oxide synthase (iNOS), reactive oxygen species (ROS), nuclear factor kappa-light-chain-enhancer of activated B cells (NF-κB), and heme oxygenase (HO-1) increase adipocyte lipolysis and systemic insulin resistance by stimulating the release of free fatty acids from adipose tissue into the blood stream, which acts on the muscle and liver [4].

The gut microbiome and adipose tissue responses play an essential role in the pathogenesis of alcohol liver disease. The mechanism between adipose tissue and alcohol consumption is yet to be answered.

2. Adipose tissue

An obese person can have up to 80 L volume of adipose tissue, which contains about 24 L volume of biologically active adipose tissue [7, 8]. The factors that affect the distribution and volume of adipose tissue mainly vary by gender and location. For example, body fat is found more in women than in men. Similarly people from southeast Asia have less body fat compared to white people of identical body mass index (BMI) [9].

Depending upon the anatomy, adipose tissue is classified as follows:

- Visceral adipose tissue (VAT)
- Subcutaneous adipose tissue (SAT)

Visceral adipose tissue corresponds with insulin resistance and diabetes mellitus [10].

2.1 What does adipose tissue composed of?

Adipocytes are considered to be the building blocks of adipose tissue. Adipocyte stores energy from non-esterified fatty acids (NEFA) and esterification of triglyceride [11]. Lipotoxicity refers to as uptake of circulating lipids, which prevents accumulation of NEFA in the organs [12]. There are various processes that take place in adipose tissue which are controlled by hormonal pathways and are useful for metabolic demand [13]:

- Hydrolysis of triglycerides (lipolysis) takes place during fasting or exercise.
- Synthesis of triglyceride (lipogenesis) takes place during fed state.

2.2 Which cytokines are released by adipocytes?

Adipose tissue secretes adipokines that play a central role in metabolism of energy. The secretion of adipokines can be altered due to obesity and insulin resistance. Out of several adipokines, leptin, adiponectin, and resistin are the primary ones that are responsible for insulin resistance as well as in ALD [14].

2.3 Different kind of adipokines:

2.3.1 Leptin

Leptin receptor is located in numerous tissues, which controls expenditure of energy, food consumption, lipolysis, fatty acid oxidation, lipogenesis, and insulin sensitivity signifying as a paracrine and autocrine hormonal function [15]. It also helps in enhancing the release of a TNF-α by Kupffer cells [16].

2.3.2 Adiponectin

Adiponectin has a significant role in insulin sensitizing by altering the signaling pathway of AMPK and metabolism of glucose and fatty acid oxidation in tissues. It is also responsible for adiopogenesis, prevention of ectopic fat storage and decline in Kupffer cell activation [14, 16]. The onset of chronic exposure to ethanol can lead to the disruption of adiponectin which is proven to contribute toward the imbalance of pro-inflammatory pathways [3]. A preventive study was performed on the mice along with the treatment of adiponectin and chronic ethanol exposure and signifies the prevention of the liver injury indicating the decrease in both steatosis and TNF-α expression in the liver [17]. Though the mechanism of the therapeutic adiponectin is not well understood, the hypothesis suggests the vital role of a adiponectin in decreasing steatosis which is related to glucose and lipid homeostasis [3].

2.3.3 Resistin

Resistin can acquire insulin resistance and regulates food intake, thus acting as an antagonist to adiponectin [18]. Resistin, a 12.5-kDa polypeptide, is secreted by white adipose tissue in female [19]. In human, resistin gene is mainly found in the bone marrow and lung with untraceable levels in adipose tissue [20]. Resistin gene expression was provoked during adipocyte differentiation [21]. Thus, serum resistin can act as a powerful diagnostic marker to access the severity of liver disease and patient with clinical complications [22].

2.3.4 Omentin

Omentin secretion increases insulin sensitivity in adipocytes [16]. It is mainly secreted from the stromal vascular fraction of adipose tissue which enhances glucose uptake mainly activated by insulin [23]. The concentration of omentin was increased in portal vein which is a consistent marker for ALD [24].

2.3.5 Chemerin

Chemerin helps pre-adipocyte differentiation and contributes to immune cell trafficking. It is also proven to increase the sensitivity of insulin as well as provides anti-inflammatory effects on endothelium immune cell [25].

2.4 The role of non-adipocytes

Non-adipocyte cells are present in a considerable amount of overall cellularity of the adipose tissue. They include cells from perivascular, endothelium, immune, and stem cells. These clusters of cells are known as stromal vascular fraction (SVF) [14].

2.4.1 Macrophages as inflammatory mediators

Macrophages make up the majority of the resident immune cells in the adipose tissue [26]. The systemic insulin resistance and inflammation are linked with increased macrophage infiltration into the adipose tissue indicating M1 pro-inflammatory state [27]. "Crown-like structure" is formed where macrophages present in adipose tissue encircle dying adipocytes [28]. Adiponectin suppresses macrophage activity using several ways; one of them is to prevent proliferation of myelomonocytic progenitor cells. This reduces the upregulation of endothelial adhesion molecules in response to cytokine production by macrophages [3].

There are other immune cells like B cells, T cells, and dendritic cells which contribute to the obesity-related inflammation. Dendritic cell in particular promotes $CD4^+$ T helper cells to activate macrophage recruitment [29]. Neutrophils are seen in lean and obese individuals, which are primary defense cells in a high-fructose diet mice model [30]. Thus, cytokine expression in adipose tissue is predominately from SVF, while in case of obese individuals, there is an increased expression of cytokines [31, 32]. Studies suggested the important link between the adiponectin and IL-10, the two main critical anti-inflammatory mediators. For instance, adiponectin stimulates IL-10 mRNA and protein expression in RAW264.7 macrophages. In the same cells, gAcrp-mediated desensitization to LPS is prevented due to the immunoneutralization of IL-10 [3]. HO-1 shows antiproliferative, anti-inflammatory, and anti-apoptotic properties. HO-1 is considered as a vital downstream mediator of the anti-inflammatory effects of IL-10 in macrophages [33].

3. What is gut microbiota comprised of?

The human gut contains more than 400 different species, comprising of four major bacterial families that play important roles like defining the physiology of the host [34]. The majority of mammalian gut microbiota belongs to the two bacterial phyla, the gram-negative *Bacteroidetes* and the gram-positive *Firmicutes*, which play a major role in the maintenance of normal health condition, metabolism, and disease. Mainly four major families play an important role, an dthey are comprised of:

- *Bacteroidetes*
- *Firmicutes*
- *Actinobacteria*
- *Proteobacteria*

Proximal two thirds of the small intestine and stomach contain less number of microbes in the range of 10^0–10^4 cfu/ml due to acidic pH. The ileum contains more diverse microflora and higher bacterial strains from 10^7 to 10^8 cfu/ml. Most amounts of species of obligate anaerobe reside in the colon due to a low oxidation-reduction potential of the colon. Thus, a subsequent increase in microbes from the stomach to colon has been observed, as the human gastrointestinal tract pH has shown an increase from the stomach (pH 2.0) to duodenum, jejunum, ileum, and colon (pH 5.0–7.0) [35].

Bacteroidetes contain variety of enzymes like hydrolase, dehydrogenase, and dehydroxylase that play a major role in the biotransformation of bile acids. *Firmicutes* play an important role in the energy extraction from undigested carbohydrates in the form of production of short-chain fatty acids [36]. Far from being a static ecosystem, the content of this phylum radially shifts in the response to change in host adiposity and nutrient uptake [37].

Changes in the intake of diet clearly affect composition of an individual's gut microbiota and its body physiology [38]. Complex carbohydrates are metabolized by the colonic microorganism. *Bifidobacteria* convert complex carbohydrates into oligosaccharides and monosaccharide, further fermenting into the short-chain fatty acid end products like acetate, propionate, and butyrate. Colon absorbs SCFA, where butyrate provides energy for colonic epithelial cells; acetate and propionate migrate to the liver and other peripheral organs, where they act as substrates for gluconeogenesis and lipogenesis [39].

3.1 Gut microflora in well-being, metabolism, and disease

3.1.1 How does gut microflora gets affected in nonalcoholic fatty liver disease?

Nonalcoholic fatty liver disease is the liver disorder whose pathogenesis is not well understood due to the portal system interaction with the intestinal lumen and liver. Therefore, it is considered that gut microbiome plays an important role in the pathogenesis of NAFLD. Also, diet has a potential to modify the gut microbiome and several metabolic pathways. Thus, the combination of diet, gut, and liver associates directly with the progression of NAFLD or T2D. Most of the diabetic patients are diagnosed with high blood glucose levels in context with insulin resistance and insulin deficiency.

Westernized diet and pattern of eating are the main driving forces for the increased prevalence of insulin resistance and increased obesity. Studies have suggested that the diet rich in saturated fats are directly proportional to weight gain, insulin resistance, and hyperlipidemia in humans and animal models [40]. In addition, diet specifically high in sugars like fructose and sucrose has contributed to the metabolic alterations in animal models resulting in weight gain hyperlipidemia and hypertension [41]. An overconsumption of fructose hampers glycolysis and glucose uptake pathways in the liver. This leads to an enhanced rate of de novo lipogenesis and triacylglycerol synthesis leading to insulin resistance through fructose catabolism.

Increased activity of the inflammatory pathways is a very important mechanism for insulin resistance. An increase in the activity of the nuclear factor kB (NF-kB) pathway and the maintenance of a subacute inflammatory state are associated with obesity. These cytokines and chemokine activate intracellular pathways which promote the development of T2D [42]. Pattern recognition receptors (PRRs) play an important role for identification of commensals versus pathogenic microbes, which reside in the gastrointestinal tract. TLR recognize extracellular patterns, whereas NOD-like receptors (NLRs) recognize intracellular (cytosolic) pathogen Associated molecular patterns (PAMPs) [43].

TLRs, extracellular (innate) pattern recognition receptors, are expressed nearly on all the cell types. In total, 13 different TLRs are present in human genome, which remain specific for unique class of PAMPs. Among the TLRs, TLR2 and TLR4 are considered to be vital for the pathogenesis of insulin resistance and diabetes in both clinical and experimental conditions. TLR2 specifically binds to peptidoglycan (gram-positive bacteria), and TLR4 binds to lipopolysaccharide (gram-negative bacteria) [43]. High-fat or high carbohydrate food intake increases the concentration of plasma LPS levels and LPS binding protein, which increases the expression of TLR2 and TLR4 at mRNA and protein level [44]. The study has also shown that the absence of TLR4 protects against the detrimental effects of obesity and lipids on the insulin resistance [44]. A study on TLR4 null mice demonstrated a reduced adiposity and hepatic steatosis compared with the wild-type control when fed on high fat diet (HFD) [45].

NLRs are intracellular or cytoplasmic pattern recognition receptors, which exhibit specificity toward one or more PAMPs. In gastrointestinal epithelial cells, nucleotide-binding oligomerization domain (NOD) is mainly characterized by NLRs. Caspase activation and recruitment domain (CARD) is unique for each NOD protein.

- NOD1 (CARD 4): senses peptidoglycan contents in gram-negative bacteria specifically meso-diaminopimelic acid (meso-DAP)

- NOD2 (CARD 15): senses muramyl dipeptide, the common molecular motif both in gram-positive and gram-negative bacteria.

NOD1 and NOD2 are essential since they were the first NLRs reported as potential sensors of bacterial components. It has been reported that NOD1 and NOD2 are also involved in high fat diet induced-inflammation and insulin intolerance [46]. NOD1 agonist causes inflammation and insulin resistance in a primary hepatocytes of the wild-type mice, but this effect was absent in NOD1 knockout mice [47].

The downstream pathway that follows after the engagement of NLRs and TLRs with their respective ligands leads to the activation of NF-kB-mediated inflammatory pathways through adaptor protein MyD88 and secretes the major pro-inflammatory cytokines like TNF-α and IL-6. Pro-inflammatory cytokines phosphorylate the serine/threonine residue of insulin and downregulate the insulin signaling pathway, which finally leads to the insulin resistance and occurrence of T2D [48]. In vivo studies in mice have shown that the gut tight junction between the cells loosens up when the population of *Bifidobacteria* is decreased. These loose junctions increase the gut permeability and allow lipopolysaccharide present in microbes to pass through the gut epithelial resulting into metabolic endotoxemia causing a low-grade inflammation which is responsible to induce a metabolic disorder including the insulin resistance [49].

Increased body weight with other metabolic phenotypes was observed in the germ-free mice who were fed with either low-fat mouse chow or with different levels of saturated fat and fruits along with vegetables in different groups [50]. In another study, group of mice developed hyperglycemia and high plasma concentration of pro-inflammatory cytokines when HFD was induced. Hyperglycemia resulted in hepatic macro-vesicular steatosis, elevated hepatic triglycerides, and de novo lipogenesis [51].

When an adult germ-free C57BL/6 mouse was orally fed with normal microbiota harvested from the distal intestine of any normal animals, they developed 60% increase in body fat content with insulin resistance. Fasting-induced adipocyte factor (FIAF), a circulating protein of angiopoietin, is essential for the microbiota-induced deposition of triglycerides in adipocytes [52]. Deficiency of choline is usually liked with NAFLD and nonalcoholic steatohepatitis (NASH) [53].

The above-mentioned examples show the significance of the environment and genetic factors in correlation with the liver diseases.

3.1.2 How does a whole body responds to alcoholic liver disease?

The liver is a vital organ of the body, as it metabolizes alcohol in three different ways as follows:

- By the use of an enzyme alcohol dehydrogenase (ADH)
- By the use of CYP2E1
- By the use of mitochondrial catalase

ADH and CYP2E1 are two significant ways through which alcohol gets converted into acetaldehyde; ADH is used when the consumption of alcohol is limited, while on the consumption of an excess alcohol, CYP2E1 metabolism plays a role [54]. ADH is not only present in the liver but, it also is expressed in the gastric mucosa. It is an assumption that people with lower gastric ADH are more prone to the alcoholic liver disease [55].

Alcoholic liver disease includes various stages like alcoholic hepatitis, steatosis, steatohepatitis, fibrosis, cirrhosis, and hepatocellular carcinoma. Alcohol consumption, diet, nutrition, and genetics determine the severity and prognosis of ALD. Morbidity and mortality remain higher in the liver cirrhosis than in benign liver disease (i.e., liver steatosis) [54]. Twenty percent of the patients with simple steatosis with continuous abuse can develop fibrosis within a period of 10 years [56]. In an absence of alcohol for a few weeks, simple steatosis is reversible, while a fibrogenic process of steatohepatitis can induce cirrhosis. Human trials on reversing the steatohepatitis for the treatment of chronic hepatitis C and NASH are well documented [57].

Oxidative stress mainly occurs due to CYP2E1 accompanied along with the shortage of antioxidants in the hepatocytes and an altered inflammatory cytokines [58]. It has been known that changes in the lipid metabolism and adipose tissue will also enhance the process of liver injury [59]. Genetics of an individual is also another factor that is taken into account for the susceptibility of alcoholism. Lately correlations between the genetic polymorphism of alcoholic metabolizing enzymes and ALD have shown a significant association [60]. Family studies in Asian population have shown association of the following two genes in particular with ALD [61, 62].

- Alcohol dehydrogenase ADH1B*1 allele: responsible for increase in alcohol dependence
- Alcohol dehydrogenase ADH2B*2 allele: responsible for decrease in alcohol dependence

Diet is also one of the significant factors affecting the structure and functionality of gut microbiota. Alcohol and its degradation products can contribute toward the gut dysbiosis [63]. Patients with ALD have shown decrease in commensal groups like *Roseburia*, *Faecalibacterium*, *Blautia*, and *Bacteroides*, while increase in *Proteobacteria* and *Bacilli* resulting in an increased gut permeability, tight junction barrier dysfunctioning, and inflammation [64, 65]. One of the proposed mechanisms is the direct interaction of gut and endotoxins from the liver via hepatic artery, as well as mechanism of bile acids that contributes toward ALD [66], although the mechanism of the latter interaction is yet to be elucidated.

Due to an exposure of alcohol, intestinal microbiome is getting affected by causing bacterial (gram negative) overgrowth in animal models and humans. Particularly the genus *Lactobacillus* is on a lower side due to the onset of chronic alcohol consumption [67]. It has been recently demonstrated that supplementing saturated long-chain fatty acid with commensal *Lactobacilli* stabilizes the intestinal gut barrier and tight junction barrier in ethanol-induced liver disease in mice [68]. NOD2 is mainly responsible for increasing bacterial peritonitis and bacterascites in cirrhosis, which primarily affects the survival [69]. PAMPs or damage-associated molecular patterns (DAMPs) are recognized by inflammasomes and activate the pro-inflammatory cytokines such as pro-interleukin (IL-1, IL-18) [70]. Chemokine (C-C motif) ligand causes inflammation in colon due to intestinal dysbiosis [71]. TNF-receptor-1 (TNFR-1) present on the intestinal epithelial cells are crucial mediator for ALD and also cause an intestinal barrier dysbiosis [72]. Thus, inflammation can lead to intestinal permeability, which is associated with the translocation of microbial products to TLRs in the liver, which is related to aggravated hepatic steatosis.

4. Role of immune system in intestinal membrane

Maintaining the balance and symbiotic relation between the immune system and host intestinal microbiome is a very important aspect. This is because they maintain a balance of an immune system by restricting the overgrowth of pathogenic microbiota, as well as the bacteria that reaches the intestinal barriers, chemical barriers, and physical barriers [73]. Innate signaling by MyD88 in T cells directs IgA-mediated microbiota to promote the healthy gut. In IgA-deficient mice, it has been observed that TLR-5 and host protein programmed cell death 1 (PD1) regulate the modulation of IgA homeostasis by differentiating B cells into IgA producing antibodies [74, 75]. The importance of IgA in the microbiota composition in chronic liver disease is yet to be studied.

In liver cirrhosis patient, buccal origin microbes were found in intestine, taxonomically signifying the translocation or invasion from mouth to intestine. Simultaneously these patients also observed to have compromised innate immune system, reduced bile flow and impaired AMP production [76, 77]. The production of AMP is mainly regulated by the gut microbiota that includes defensins, C-type lectins (Reg3b and Reg3g), ribonucleases, and S100 proteins, which rapidly inactivate microbes [78]. In MYD88-deficient mice, NOD2 altered AMP production, which was closely marked [79, 80]. Chronic alcohol administration results in decreased expression of the intestinal C-type lectins in mice, and similar results were observed in the duodenum [81, 82].

Mucin is secreted by the goblet cells which are glycosylated and accountable for the construction of the inner and outer layer of mucus. In mice and humans, mainly mucin-2 is responsible for the mucus layer formation. Upon interaction with the lectin, they are responsible for bacterial composition of the host that promotes formation of glycosidase and metabolic enzymes which are used as a source of energy [83]. Innate immune system is activated to maintain the intestinal homeostasis in the absence of mucin-2. An experiment in the mucin-2-deficient mice demonstrated higher expression of antimicrobial proteins and protected the intestinal barrier from bacterial overgrowth and dysbiosis. This interconnection between the different intestinal defense layers and microbiota helps in decreasing ALD [81].

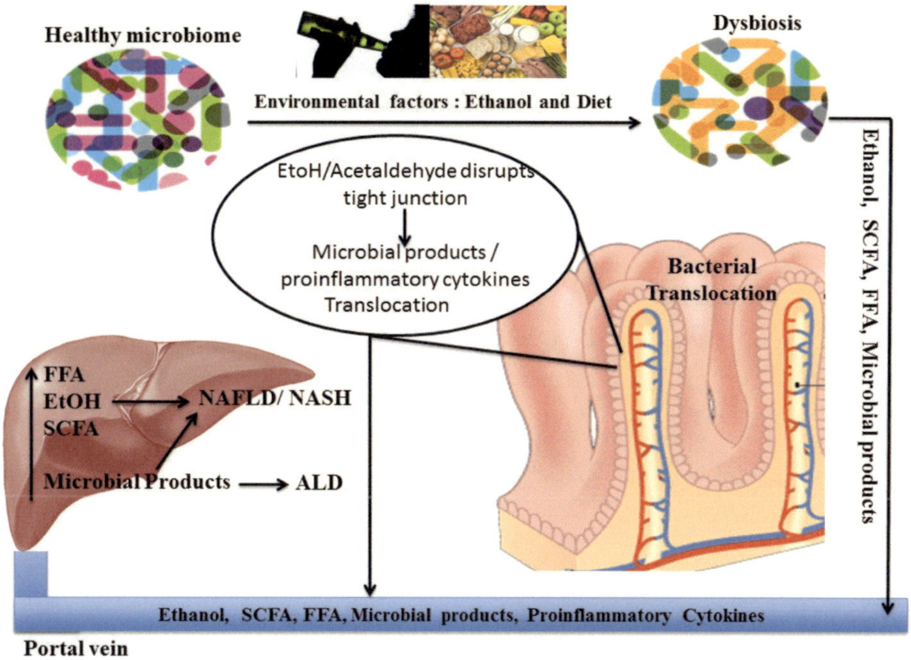

Figure 1.
Effect of microbiome dysbiosis on liver disease.

Interestingly, there is no single assigned bacterial species that marks the beginning or development of the liver disease. It is always marked by an increased percentage of gram-negative bacteria especially *Proteobacteria* which is known for accelerating cholestatic liver fibrosis [84]. To study the importance of the intestinal microbiota for chronic liver disease, liver fibrosis was induced into the germ-free mice model via the administration of thioacetamide in the drinking water. As a result in comparison to conventional mice, germ-free mice showed elevated liver fibrosis [85].

Ethanol consumptions lead to the elevation of lipopolysaccharide and endotoxin in the portal blood circulation that sensitizes Kupffer cells to activate the inflammatory mediators like TNF-α, IL6, and ROS. Another factor that facilitates the liver disease is the loss of anti-inflammatory mediators. A study has shown IL-10 deficient mice to be more sensitive to ethanol liver injury [3]. The alterations in the intestinal microbiota composition are significant for the pathogenesis of chronic liver disease which is demonstrated and briefed in **Figure 1**.

5. Effect of alcohol on liver and adipose tissue

The energy value of alcohol is equal to those of other nutrients, so when the alcohol consumption is increased, the overall calorie intake excessed the expenditure of energy, which leads to adiposity [86]. It has been established that chronic cirrhosis patient shifts toward the lipid oxidation instead of carbohydrate as fuel to meet the energy requirements which in turn reduces the overall fat mass in an individual [87]. Thus, malnutrition with low adipose skeletal muscle mass is a symptom for an advancement of the liver disease [88]. Alterations in the body mass may also depend on the type of drinking pattern; for instance, a person drinking beer or spirits gains more body mass than wine consumption [89]. Thus, excess alcohol

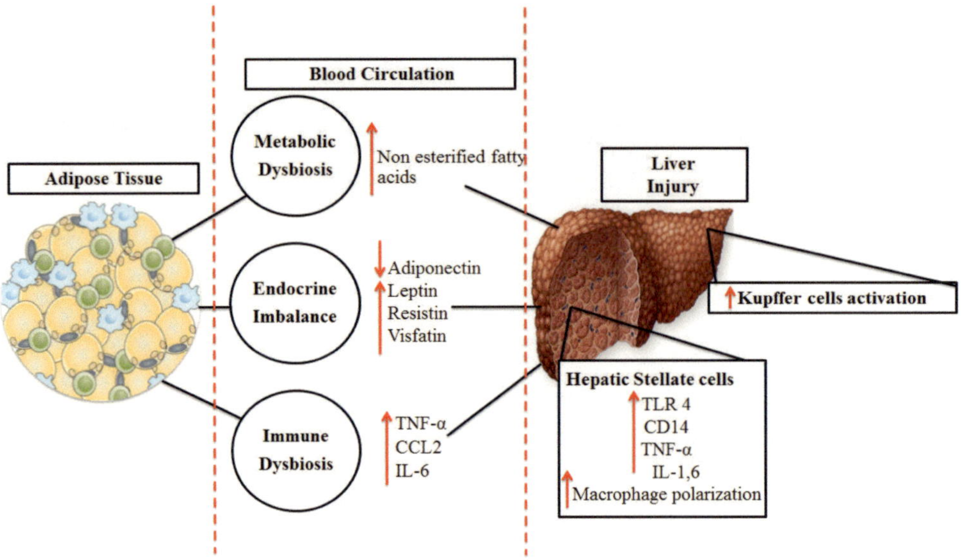

Figure 2.
Association of adipose tissue in alcoholism due to metabolic, endocrine, and immune dysbiosis.

intake increases the amount of visceral adipose tissue as compared to the changes observed in case of obesity [90].

In vivo mice experimental alcoholic model has shown the significant increase in the number of adipocyte death in white adipose tissue. The mechanism for death of adipocytes involves interaction between CYP2E1, BH3-an interaction domain agonist for death (BID) and C1Q complement pathway. As sequence, these interaction lead to adipose tissue inflammation, insulin resistance, lipolysis, NEFA and release of proinflammatory cytokines [91]. Hence, increase in uptake of fatty acids in the adipose tissue will lead to an increase in hypertrophy, hypoxia, and inflammation ultimately leading to the cell death [92]. However, alcohol uptake in the moderation has been associated with insulin sensitivity [93]. Thus, acute or chronic alcohol consumption is associated with metabolic, endocrine, and immune dysbiosis as shown in **Figure 2**.

5.1 Influence of alcohol on metabolic dysbiosis

Metabolically, an increase of NEFA is seen in ALD patients [94]. Increase in NEFA depends on the increase in expression of adipose triglyceride lipase (ATGL) but is independent of lipase [95]. Lipolysis is particularly marked by acute alcoholic hepatitis (AAH), but it may decrease during the advanced cirrhosis. The molecular mechanism that leads to lipolysis with excess ethanol consumption is not clearly understood; the possible primary factor may be the ethanol-mediated insulin resistance. Contradicting effect is seen with the use of catecholamine, which may reduce lipolysis or remain unchanged [96]. Consequently, higher level of circulating NEFA shows reduced capacity of the adipose tissue to esterify alcohol and store up free fatty acid [97]. Further these unsaturated fatty acids are delivered to the liver which contributes to hepatic steatosis as they get converted to triglyceride [98]. c-Jun N-terminal kinase (JNK) pathway triggers the hepatocyte apoptosis by increase in number of saturated fatty acids with enhanced hepatotoxic effect [99]. Hepatic de novo lipogenesis increases due to the transcription of sterol regulatory

Adipokine	In vivo model (mouse and human)	Acute alcoholic model	Chronic alcoholic model	Reference
Leptin	In both models	↓	↓	[102]
Adiponectin* (high fat diet and alcohol)	In human model	↑	↑	[103]
	In mouse model	↑	↑	[104]
Visfatin	In both models	↑	↑	[105]
Omentin	In human model	↑	↑	[24]
Chemerin	In human model	↑	↑ Chronic alcoholic patient	[106]
			↓ Cirrhosis patient	[107]

**Adiponectin data are in contrast with the observation in individual with obesity and metabolic syndrome due to changes in liver function while affecting the bile obstruction.*

Table 1.
The changes in adipokines in mouse and human models with severity of alcohol abuse.

element-binding protein 1 (*Srebf1*) [100]. The mechanism that follows in hepatocytes on increase in NEFA activates the hepatic stellate cells (HSCs) which lead to the deposition of collagen and fibrosis, which in turn exerts the inflammatory pathway through stimulation of NF-κB and the activation of Kupffer cells and myeloid cells stimulating cytokine release [101].

5.2 Endocrine imbalance due to consumption of alcohol

Acute or chronic alcohol intake has an important difference in both animal and human models with respect to the endocrine aspect as shown in **Table 1**.

Due to the change in an endocrine function, the liver fibrosis takes place by promoting HSC activation [108]. Leptin contributes to the activation of TNF-alpha and the Kupffer cells, thereby causing hepatic inflammation by stimulating CCL2 release from HSCs [109]. The administration of adiponectin and recombinant adiponectin in ethanol-fed mice reduced the circulating NEFA level as well as decreased weight loss, steatosis, and hepatic inflammation due to the inhibition of Kupffer cell sensitivity toward LPS [67].

5.3 Immune dysbiosis due to alcohol intake

Oxidative stress due to the consumption of alcohol leads to adipose tissue hypoxia which in turn increases the expression of TNF-α, CCL2, IL-6, infiltration of macrophages, and expression of $CD4^+$ T cells and dendritic cells in the adipose tissue [110]. The secretion of pro-inflammatory cytokines alters the hepatic immunology via hepatic inflammation affecting the role of parenchymal and non-parenchymal liver cells. TNF-α activation triggers ALD pathogenesis, which induces apoptosis through the activation of JNK and NFκB pathways [111]. A protective mechanism of the hepatocytes is exerted by IL-6 through promoting the hepatic survival, proliferation, and improved hepatic steatosis [112]. Nevertheless, an excessive exposure of IL-6 can lead to the liver carcinogenesis [113]. In CCL2 knockout mice, there is a reduced level of hepatic inflammation, proving CCL2 to not play any protective role in hepatic inflammation [114]. The role of CCL2 is much more clear as an inflammatory factor through an insulin signaling in NASH, but its role in ALD is yet to be determined [115].

5.4 Role of microRNA

Exosomes that contain small biologically active but noncoding RNA, i.e., microRNA (miRNA), are released by adipocytes which regulate various intracellular processes. These miRNAs are able to temper the distant tissues and organs representing the alteration between adipose tissue and liver function as well as immune responses [116]. In an animal model, miRNA-122 and miRNA-192 expressions are elevated in the ALD, while miRNA-155 expression is increased in the adipose tissues in particular, which contributes to the hepatic steatosis and fibrosis [117].

6. Conclusion

Chronic alcohol consumption not only disturbs the metabolism of whole body but also has a prominent effect on the function of gut microbiota and adipose tissue. These alterations have direct as well as indirect effects on the liver functions, which contribute to the advancement of ALD. Cessation of alcohol intake can quickly reverse inflammatory reaction in the adipose tissue and halt the progression of ALD. In addition to that, pharmacological treatment can also help to improve ALD. There is a significant overlapping in an alteration of the adipose tissue between obesity, NAFLD, and ALD mechanism. The physicians who are dealing with patients of ALD should keep an eye on the adipose tissue dysfunction and its effect on the liver and consider the therapeutic treatment accordingly. Understanding the fundamental mechanism of the alcohol and metabolic syndrome in the pathogenesis of liver disease will help in pursuing an effective treatment for liver diseases.

Author details

Dhara Patel and Palash Mandal*
Department of Biological Sciences, P.D. Patel Institute of Applied Sciences, Charotar University of Science and Technology, Anand, Gujarat, India

*Address all correspondence to: palashmandal.bio@charusat.ac.in

References

[1] Rehm J, Samokhvalov AV, Shield KD. Global burden of alcoholic liver diseases. Journal of Hepatology. 2013;**59**:160-168. DOI: 10.1016/j.jhep.2013.03.007

[2] O'Shea RS, Dasarathy S, McCullough AJ, Practice Guideline Committee of the American Association for the Study of Liver Diseases, Practice Parameters Committee of the American College of Gastroenterology. Alcoholic liver disease. Hepatology. 2010;**51**: 307-328. DOI: 10.1002/hep.23258

[3] Mandal P, Park P-H, McMullen MR, Pratt BT, Nagy LE. The anti-inflammatory effects of adiponectin are mediated via a heme oxygenase-1-dependent pathway in rat Kupffer cells. Hepatology. 2010;**51**:1420-1429. DOI: 10.1002/hep.23427

[4] Steiner J, Lang C. Alcohol, adipose tissue and lipid dysregulation. Biomolecules. 2017;**7**:16. DOI: 10.3390/biom7010016

[5] Sun X, Tang Y, Tan X, Li Q, Zhong W, Sun X, et al. Activation of peroxisome proliferator-activated receptor-γ by rosiglitazone improves lipid homeostasis at the adipose tissue-liver axis in ethanol-fed mice. American Journal of Physiology. Gastrointestinal and Liver Physiology. 2012;**302**:G548-G557. DOI: 10.1152/ajpgi.00342.2011

[6] Zhang W, Zhong W, Sun X, Sun Q, Tan X, Li Q, et al. Visceral white adipose tissue is susceptible to alcohol-induced lipodystrophy in rats: Role of acetaldehyde. Alcoholism, Clinical and Experimental Research. 2015;**39**: 416-423. DOI: 10.1111/acer.12646

[7] Molina DK, DiMaio VJM. Normal organ weights in women. The American Journal of Forensic Medicine and Pathology. 2015;**36**:176-181. DOI: 10.1097/PAF.0000000000000174

[8] Molina DK, DiMaio VJM. Normal organ weights in men. The American Journal of Forensic Medicine and Pathology. 2012;**33**:368-372. DOI: 10.1097/PAF.0b013e31823d29ad

[9] Nazare J-A, Smith JD, Borel A-L, Haffner SM, Balkau B, Ross R, et al. Ethnic influences on the relations between abdominal subcutaneous and visceral adiposity, liver fat, and cardiometabolic risk profile: The international study of prediction of intra-abdominal adiposity and its relationship with cardiometabolic risk/intra-abdominal adiposity. The American Journal of Clinical Nutrition. 2012;**96**:714-726. DOI: 10.3945/ajcn.112.035758

[10] Raji A, Seely EW, Arky RA, Simonson DC. Body fat distribution and insulin resistance in healthy Asian Indians and Caucasians. The Journal of Clinical Endocrinology and Metabolism. 2001;**86**:5366-5371. DOI: 10.1210/jcem.86.11.7992

[11] Rutkowski JM, Stern JH, Scherer PE. The cell biology of fat expansion. The Journal of Cell Biology. 2015;**208**:501-512. DOI: 10.1083/jcb.201409063

[12] Cusi K. Role of obesity and lipotoxicity in the development of nonalcoholic steatohepatitis: Pathophysiology and clinical implications. Gastroenterology. 2012;**142**:711-725. DOI: 10.1053/j.gastro.2012.02.003

[13] Nielsen TS, Jessen N, Jorgensen JOL, Moller N, Lund S. Dissecting adipose tissue lipolysis: Molecular regulation and implications for metabolic disease. Journal of Molecular Endocrinology. 2014;**52**:R199-R222. DOI: 10.1530/JME-13-0277

[14] Patel D, Patel F, Mandal P. Potential molecular mechanism of

probiotics in alcoholic liver disease. Journal of Alcoholism and Drug Dependence. 2017;**5**:1-11. DOI: 10.4172/2329-6488.1000278

[15] Stern JH, Rutkowski JM, Scherer PE. Adiponectin, leptin, and fatty acids in the maintenance of metabolic homeostasis through adipose tissue crosstalk. Cell Metabolism. 2016;**23**: 770-784. DOI: 10.1016/j.cmet.2016.04.011

[16] Parker R, Kim S-J, Gao B. Alcohol, adipose tissue and liver disease: Mechanistic links and clinical considerations. Nature Reviews. Gastroenterology & Hepatology. 2017;**15**:50-59. DOI: 10.1038/nrgastro.2017.116

[17] Xu A, Wang Y, Keshaw H, Xu LY, Lam KSL, Cooper GJS. The fat-derived hormone adiponectin alleviates alcoholic and nonalcoholic fatty liver diseases in mice. The Journal of Clinical Investigation. 2003;**112**:91-100. DOI: 10.1172/JCI17797

[18] Vázquez MJ, González CR, Varela L, Lage R, Tovar S, Sangiao-Alvarellos S, et al. Central resistin regulates hypothalamic and peripheral lipid metabolism in a nutritional-dependent fashion. Endocrinology. 2008;**149**:4534-4543. DOI: 10.1210/en.2007-1708

[19] Pravdova E, Fickova M. Alcohol intake modulates hormonal activity of adipose tissue. Endocrine Regulations. 2006;**40**:91-104

[20] Patel L, Buckels AC, Kinghorn IJ, Murdock PR, Holbrook JD, Plumpton C, et al. Resistin is expressed in human macrophages and directly regulated by PPAR gamma activators. Biochemical and Biophysical Research Communications. 2003;**300**:472-476

[21] Steppan CM, Bailey ST, Bhat S, Brown EJ, Banerjee RR, Wright CM, et al. The hormone resistin links obesity to diabetes. Nature. 2001;**409**:307-312. DOI: 10.1038/35053000

[22] Yagmur E, Trautwein C, Gressner AM, Tacke F. Resistin serum levels are associated with insulin resistance, disease severity, clinical complications, and prognosis in patients with chronic liver diseases. The American Journal of Gastroenterology. 2006;**101**:1244-1252. DOI: 10.1111/j.1572-0241.2006.00543.x

[23] Yang R-Z, Lee M-J, Hu H, Pray J, Wu H-B, Hansen BC, et al. Identification of omentin as a novel depot-specific adipokine in human adipose tissue: Possible role in modulating insulin action. American Journal of Physiology. Endocrinology and Metabolism. 2006;**290**:E1253-E1261. DOI: 10.1152/ajpendo.00572.2004

[24] Eisinger K, Krautbauer S, Wiest R, Karrasch T, Hader Y, Scherer MN, et al. Portal vein omentin is increased in patients with liver cirrhosis but is not associated with complications of portal hypertension. European Journal of Clinical Investigation. 2013;**43**:926-932. DOI: 10.1111/eci.12122

[25] Ernst MC, Sinal CJ. Chemerin: At the crossroads of inflammation and obesity. Trends in Endocrinology and Metabolism. 2010;**21**:660-667. DOI: 10.1016/j.tem.2010.08.001

[26] Weisberg SP, McCann D, Desai M, Rosenbaum M, Leibel RL, Ferrante AW. Obesity is associated with macrophage accumulation in adipose tissue. The Journal of Clinical Investigation. 2003;**112**:1796-1808. DOI: 10.1172/JCI19246

[27] Lumeng CN, Bodzin JL, Saltiel AR. Obesity induces a phenotypic switch in adipose tissue macrophage polarization. The Journal of Clinical Investigation. 2007;**117**:175-184. DOI: 10.1172/JCI29881

[28] Lumeng CN, DelProposto JB, Westcott DJ, Saltiel AR. Phenotypic switching of adipose tissue macrophages with obesity is generated by spatiotemporal differences in macrophage subtypes. Diabetes. 2008;**57**:3239-3246. DOI: 10.2337/db08-0872

[29] Stefanovic-Racic M, Yang X, Turner MS, Mantell BS, Stolz DB, Sumpter TL, et al. Dendritic cells promote macrophage infiltration and comprise a substantial proportion of obesity-associated increases in CD11c+ cells in adipose tissue and liver. Diabetes. 2012;**61**:2330-2339. DOI: 10.2337/db11-1523

[30] Elgazar-Carmon V, Rudich A, Hadad N, Levy R. Neutrophils transiently infiltrate intra-abdominal fat early in the course of high-fat feeding. Journal of Lipid Research. 2008;**49**:1894-1903. DOI: 10.1194/jlr.M800132-JLR200

[31] Xu H, Barnes GT, Yang Q, Tan G, Yang D, Chou CJ, et al. Chronic inflammation in fat plays a crucial role in the development of obesity-related insulin resistance. The Journal of Clinical Investigation. 2003;**112**:1821-1830. DOI: 10.1172/JCI19451

[32] Fain JN. Release of interleukins and other inflammatory cytokines by human adipose tissue is enhanced in obesity and primarily due to the nonfat cells. Vitamins and Hormones. 2006;**74**:443-477. DOI: 10.1016/S0083-6729(06)74018-3

[33] Otterbein LE, Soares MP, Yamashita K, Bach FH. Heme oxygenase-1: Unleashing the protective properties of heme. Trends in Immunology. 2003;**24**:449-455

[34] Nicholson JK, Holmes E, Wilson ID. Opinion: Gut microorganisms, mammalian metabolism and personalized health care. Nature Reviews. Microbiology. 2005;**3**:431-438. DOI: 10.1038/nrmicro1152

[35] Sekirov I, Russell SL, Antunes LCM, Finlay BB. Gut microbiota in health and disease. Physiological Reviews. 2010;**90**:859-904. DOI: 10.1152/physrev.00045.2009

[36] Guarner F, Malagelada J-R. Gut flora in health and disease. Lancet. 2003;**361**:512-519. DOI: 10.1016/S0140-6736(03)12489-0

[37] Ley RE, Turnbaugh PJ, Klein S, Gordon JI. Microbial ecology: Human gut microbes associated with obesity. Nature. 2006;**444**:1022-1023. DOI: 10.1038/4441022a

[38] Flint HJ, Scott KP, Louis P, Duncan SH. The role of the gut microbiota in nutrition and health. Nature Reviews. Gastroenterology & Hepatology. 2012;**9**:577-589. DOI: 10.1038/nrgastro.2012.156

[39] Cani PD, Delzenne NM. The role of the gut microbiota in energy metabolism and metabolic disease. Current Pharmaceutical Design. 2009;**15**:1546-1558

[40] Kootte RS, Vrieze A, Holleman F, Dallinga-Thie GM, Zoetendal EG, de Vos WM, et al. The therapeutic potential of manipulating gut microbiota in obesity and type 2 diabetes mellitus. Diabetes, Obesity and Metabolism. 2012;**14**:112-120. DOI: 10.1111/j.1463-1326.2011.01483.x

[41] Vrieze A, Holleman F, Zoetendal EG, de Vos WM, Hoekstra JBL, Nieuwdorp M. The environment within: How gut microbiota may influence metabolism and body composition. Diabetologia. 2010;**53**:606-613. DOI: 10.1007/s00125-010-1662-7

[42] Shoelson SE, Lee J, Goldfine AB. Inflammation and insulin resistance.

The Journal of Clinical Investigation. 2006;**116**:1793-1801. DOI: 10.1172/JCI29069

[43] Takeuchi O, Akira S. Pattern recognition receptors and inflammation. Cell. 2010;**140**:805-820. DOI: 10.1016/j.cell.2010.01.022

[44] Shi H, Kokoeva MV, Inouye K, Tzameli I, Yin H, Flier JS. TLR4 links innate immunity and fatty acid–induced insulin resistance. The Journal of Clinical Investigation. 2006;**116**: 3015-3025. DOI: 10.1172/JCI28898

[45] Kaushik RS, George S, Circle K, Lindblom S, Vilain S, Rosa AJM, et al. Assessment of toll-like receptors in the ileum of weanling pigs-responses to feed antibiotic chlortetracycline and gnotobiotic conditions. Journal of Clinical and Cellular Immunology. 2012;**3**:125. DOI: 10.4172/2155-9899.1000125

[46] Schertzer JD, Tamrakar AK, Magalhaes JG, Pereira S, Bilan PJ, Fullerton MD, et al. NOD1 activators link innate immunity to insulin resistance. Diabetes. 2011;**60**:2206-2215. DOI: 10.2337/db11-0004

[47] Zhao L, Hu P, Zhou Y, Purohit J, Hwang D. NOD1 activation induces proinflammatory gene expression and insulin resistance in 3T3-L1 adipocytes. American Journal Physiology Endocrinology Metabolism. 2011;**301**:E587-E598. DOI: 10.1152/ajpendo.00709.2010

[48] Basciano H, Federico L, Adeli K. Fructose, insulin resistance, and metabolic dyslipidemia. Nutrition & Metabolism (London). 2005;2:5. DOI: 10.1186/1743-7075-2-5

[49] Cani PD, Delzenne NM. Interplay between obesity and associated metabolic disorders: New insights into the gut microbiota. Current Opinion in Pharmacology. 2009;**9**:737-743. DOI: 10.1016/j.coph.2009.06.016

[50] Ridaura VK, Faith JJ, Rey FE, Cheng J, Duncan AE, Kau AL, et al. Gut microbiota from twins discordant for obesity modulate metabolism in mice. Science. 2013;**341**:1241214. DOI: 10.1126/science.1241214

[51] Turnbaugh PJ, Ley RE, Mahowald MA, Magrini V, Mardis ER, Gordon JI. An obesity-associated gut microbiome with increased capacity for energy harvest. Nature. 2006;**444**: 1027-1131. DOI: 10.1038/nature05414

[52] Backhed F, Ding H, Wang T, Hooper LV, Koh GY, Nagy A, et al. The gut microbiota as an environmental factor that regulates fat storage. Proceedings of the National Academy of Sciences. 2004;**101**:15718-15723. DOI: 10.1073/pnas.0407076101

[53] Spencer MD, Hamp TJ, Reid RW, Fischer LM, Zeisel SH, Fodor AA. Association between composition of the human gastrointestinal microbiome and development of fatty liver with choline deficiency. Gastroenterology. 2011;**140**:976-986. DOI: 10.1053/j.gastro.2010.11.049

[54] Bruha R, Dvorak K, Petrtyl J. Alcoholic liver disease. World Journal of Hepatology. 2012;**4**:81-90. DOI: 10.4254/wjh.v4.i3.81

[55] Frezza M, di Padova C, Pozzato G, Terpin M, Baraona E, Lieber CS. High blood alcohol levels in women. The New England Journal of Medicine. 1990;**322**:95-99. DOI: 10.1056/NEJM199001113220205

[56] Teli MR, James OF, Burt AD, Bennett MK, Day CP. The natural history of nonalcoholic fatty liver: A follow-up study. Hepatology. 1995;**22**:1714-1719

[57] Poynard T, Mchutchison J, Manns M, Trepo C, Lindsay K, Goodman Z, et al. Impact of pegylated interferon alfa-2b and ribavirin on

liver fibrosis in patients with chronic hepatitis C. Gastroenterology. 2002;**122**(5):1303-1313. DOI: 10.1053/gast.2002.33023

[58] Yin M, Wheeler MD, Kono H, Bradford BU, Gallucci RM, Luster MI, et al. Essential role of tumor necrosis factor alpha in alcohol-induced liver injury in mice. Gastroenterology. 1999;**117**:942-952

[59] Donohue TM. Alcohol-induced steatosis in liver cells. World Journal of Gastroenterology. 2007;**13**:4974-4978. DOI: 10.3748/WJG.V13.I37.4974

[60] Juran BD, Lazaridis KN. Concise review in mechanisms of disease genomics and complex liver disease: Challenges and opportunities. Hepatology. 2006;**44**(6):1380-1390. DOI: 10.1002/hep.21453

[61] Whitfield JB. Meta-analysis of the effects of alcohol dehydrogenase genotype on alcohol dependence and alcoholic liver disease. Alcohol and Alcoholism. 1997;**32**:613-619

[62] Thomasson HR, Crabb DW, Edenberg HJ, Li TK, Hwu HG, Chen CC, et al. Low frequency of the ADH2*2 allele among Atayal natives of Taiwan with alcohol use disorders. Alcoholism, Clinical and Experimental Research. 1994;**18**:640-643

[63] Dubinkina VB, Tyakht AV, Odintsova VY, Yarygin KS, Kovarsky BA, Pavlenko AV, et al. Links of gut microbiota composition with alcohol dependence syndrome and alcoholic liver disease. Microbiome. 2017;**5**:141. DOI: 10.1186/s40168-017-0359-2

[64] Bull-Otterson L, Feng W, Kirpich I, Wang Y, Qin X, Liu Y, et al. Metagenomic analyses of alcohol induced pathogenic alterations in the intestinal microbiome and the effect of lactobacillus rhamnosus GG treatment. PLoS One. 2013;**8**:e53028. DOI: 10.1371/journal.pone.0053028

[65] Mutlu EA, Gillevet PM, Rangwala H, Sikaroodi M, Naqvi A, Engen PA, et al. Colonic microbiome is altered in alcoholism. American Journal of Physiology. Gastrointestinal and Liver Physiology. 2012;**302**:G966-G978. DOI: 10.1152/ajpgi.00380.2011

[66] Ridlon JM, Kang D-J, Hylemon PB, Bajaj JS. Gut microbiota, cirrhosis, and alcohol regulate bile acid metabolism in the gut. Digestive Diseases. 2015;**33**: 338-345. DOI: 10.1159/000371678

[67] Leclercq S, Matamoros S, Cani PD, Neyrinck AM, Jamar F, Stärkel P, et al. Intestinal permeability, gut-bacterial dysbiosis, and behavioral markers of alcohol-dependence severity. Proceedings of the National Academy of Sciences. 2014;**111**:E4485-E4493. DOI: 10.1073/pnas.1415174111

[68] Llorente C, Schnabl B. The gut microbiota and liver disease. Cellular and Molecular Gastroenterology and Hepatology. 2015;**1**:275-284. DOI: 10.1016/j.jcmgh.2015.04.003

[69] Bruns T, Peter J, Reuken PA, Grabe DH, Schuldes SR, Brenmoehl J, et al. NOD2 gene variants are a risk factor for culture-positive spontaneous bacterial peritonitis and monomicrobial bacterascites in cirrhosis. Liver International. 2012;**32**:223-230. DOI: 10.1111/j.1478-3231.2011.02561.x

[70] Saner FH, Nowak K, Hoyer D, Rath P, Canbay A, Paul A, et al. A non-interventional study of the genetic polymorphisms of NOD2 associated with increased mortality in non-alcoholic liver transplant patients. BMC Gastroenterology. 2014;**14**:4. DOI: 10.1186/1471-230X-14-4

[71] Henao-Mejia J, Elinav E, Jin C, Hao L, Mehal WZ, Strowig T, et al. Inflammasome-mediated dysbiosis

regulates progression of NAFLD and obesity. Nature. 2012;**482**:179-185. DOI: 10.1038/nature10809

[72] Chen P, Stärkel P, Turner JR, Ho SB, Schnabl B. Dysbiosis-induced intestinal inflammation activates tumor necrosis factor receptor I and mediates alcoholic liver disease in mice. Hepatology. 2015;**61**:883-894. DOI: 10.1002/hep.27489

[73] Swidsinski A, Sydora BC, Doerffel Y, Loening-Baucke V, Vaneechoutte M, Lupicki M, et al. Viscosity gradient within the mucus layer determines the mucosal barrier function and the spatial organization of the intestinal microbiota. Inflammatory Bowel Diseases. 2007;**13**:963-970. DOI: 10.1002/ibd.20163

[74] Macpherson AJ, Gatto D, Sainsbury E, Harriman GR, Hengartner H, Zinkernagel RM. A primitive T cell-independent mechanism of intestinal mucosal IgA responses to commensal bacteria. Science. 2000;**288**:2222-2226

[75] Kawamoto S, Tran TH, Maruya M, Suzuki K, Doi Y, Tsutsui Y, et al. The inhibitory receptor PD-1 regulates IgA selection and bacterial composition in the gut. Science. 2012;**336**:485-489. DOI: 10.1126/science.1217718

[76] Teltschik Z, Wiest R, Beisner J, Nuding S, Hofmann C, Schoelmerich J, et al. Intestinal bacterial translocation in rats with cirrhosis is related to compromised paneth cell antimicrobial host defense. Hepatology. 2012;**55**:1154-1163. DOI: 10.1002/hep.24789

[77] Lu H, Wu Z, Xu W, Yang J, Chen Y, Li L. Intestinal microbiota was assessed in cirrhotic patients with hepatitis B virus infection. Microbial Ecology. 2011;**61**:693-703. DOI: 10.1007/s00248-010-9801-8

[78] Yang D, Chertov O, Oppenheim JJ. Participation of mammalian defensins and cathelicidins in anti-microbial immunity: Receptors and activities of human defensins and cathelicidin (LL-37). Journal of Leukocyte Biology. 2001;**69**:691-697

[79] Petnicki-Ocwieja T, Hrncir T, Liu Y-J, Biswas A, Hudcovic T, Tlaskalova-Hogenova H, et al. Nod2 is required for the regulation of commensal microbiota in the intestine. Proceedings of the National Academy of Sciences. 2009;**106**:15813-15818. DOI: 10.1073/pnas.0907722106

[80] Vaishnava S, Yamamoto M, Severson KM, Ruhn KA, Yu X, Koren O, et al. The antibacterial lectin RegIIIgamma promotes the spatial segregation of microbiota and host in the intestine. Science. 2011;**334**:255-258. DOI: 10.1126/science.1209791

[81] Hartmann P, Chen P, Wang HJ, Wang L, McCole DF, Brandl K, et al. Deficiency of intestinal mucin-2 ameliorates experimental alcoholic liver disease in mice. Hepatology. 2013;**58**:108-119. DOI: 10.1002/hep.26321

[82] Yan AW, Fouts DE, Brandl J, Stärkel P, Torralba M, Schott E, et al. Enteric dysbiosis associated with a mouse model of alcoholic liver disease. Hepatology. 2011;**53**:96-105. DOI: 10.1002/hep.24018

[83] Derrien M, van Passel MW, van de Bovenkamp JH, Schipper RG, de Vos WM, Dekker J. Mucin-bacterial interactions in the human oral cavity and digestive tract. Gut Microbes. 2010;**1**:254-268. DOI: 10.4161/gmic.1.4.12778

[84] De Minicis S, Rychlicki C, Agostinelli L, Saccomanno S, Candelaresi C, Trozzi L, et al. Dysbiosis contributes to fibrogenesis in the

course of chronic liver injury in mice. Hepatology. 2014;**59**:1738-1749. DOI: 10.1002/hep.26695

[85] Mazagova M, Wang L, Anfora AT, Wissmueller M, Lesley SA, Miyamoto Y, et al. Commensal microbiota is hepatoprotective and prevents liver fibrosis in mice. The FASEB Journal. 2015;**29**:1043-1055. DOI: 10.1096/fj.14-259515

[86] Mitchell MC, Herlong HF. Alcohol and nutrition: Caloric value, bioenergetics, and relationship to liver damage. Annual Review of Nutrition. 1986;**6**:457-474. DOI: 10.1146/annurev.nu.06.070186.002325

[87] Levine JA, Harris MM, Morgan MY. Energy expenditure in chronic alcohol abuse. European Journal of Clinical Investigation. 2000;**30**:779-786

[88] Pirlich M, Schutz T, Spachos T, Ertl S, Weis M, Lochs H, et al. Bioelectrical impedance analysis is a useful bedside technique to assess malnutrition in cirrhotic patients with and without ascites. Hepatology. 2000;**32**:1208-1215. DOI: 10.1053/jhep.2000.20524

[89] Sayon-Orea C, Bes-Rastrollo M, Nuñez-Cordoba JM, Basterra-Gortari FJ, Beunza JJ, Martinez-Gonzalez MA. Type of alcoholic beverage and incidence of overweight/obesity in a Mediterranean cohort: The SUN project. Nutrition. 2011;**27**:802-808. DOI: 10.1016/j.nut.2010.08.023

[90] Molenaar EA, Massaro JM, Jacques PF, Pou KM, Ellison RC, Hoffmann U, et al. Association of lifestyle factors with abdominal subcutaneous and visceral adiposity: The Framingham Heart Study. Diabetes Care. 2009;**32**: 505-510. DOI: 10.2337/dc08-1382

[91] Sebastian BM, Roychowdhury S, Tang H, Hillian AD, Feldstein AE, Stahl GL, et al. Identification of a cytochromeP4502E1/bid/C1q-dependent axis mediating inflammation in adipose tissue after chronic ethanol feeding to mice. The Journal of Biological Chemistry. 2011;**286**:35989-35997. DOI: 10.1074/jbc.M111.254201

[92] Sun K, Kusminski CM, Scherer PE. Adipose tissue remodeling and obesity. The Journal of Clinical Investigation. 2011;**121**:2094-2101. DOI: 10.1172/JCI45887

[93] Goude D, Fagerberg B, Hulthe J, AIR Study Group. Alcohol consumption, the metabolic syndrome and insulin resistance in 58-year-old clinically healthy men (AIR study). Clinical Science (London, England). 2002;**102**:345-352. DOI: 10.1042/CS1020345

[94] Rachakonda V, Gabbert C, Raina A, Li H, Malik S, DeLany JP, et al. Stratification of risk of death in severe acute alcoholic hepatitis using a panel of adipokines and cytokines. Alcoholism, Clinical and Experimental Research. 2014;**38**:2712-2721. DOI: 10.1111/acer.12558

[95] Zhong W, Zhao Y, Tang Y, Wei X, Shi X, Sun W, et al. Chronic alcohol exposure stimulates adipose tissue lipolysis in mice. The American Journal of Pathology. 2012;**180**:998-1007. DOI: 10.1016/j.ajpath.2011.11.017

[96] Kang L, Nagy LE. Chronic ethanol feeding suppresses beta-adrenergic receptor-stimulated lipolysis in adipocytes isolated from epididymal fat. Endocrinology. 2006;**147**:4330-4338. DOI: 10.1210/en.2006-0120

[97] Liangpunsakul S, Bennett R, Westerhold C, Ross RA, Crabb DW, Lai X, et al. Increasing serum pre-adipocyte factor-1 (Pref-1) correlates with decreased body fat, increased free fatty acids, and level of recent alcohol

consumption in excessive alcohol drinkers. Alcohol. 2014;**48**:795-800. DOI: 10.1016/j.alcohol.2014.07.013

[98] Wei X, Shi X, Zhong W, Zhao Y, Tang Y, Sun W, et al. Chronic alcohol exposure disturbs lipid homeostasis at the adipose tissue-liver axis in mice: Analysis of triacylglycerols using high-resolution mass spectrometry in combination with In vivo metabolite deuterium labeling. PLoS One. 2013;**8**:e55382. DOI: 10.1371/journal.pone.0055382

[99] Malhi H, Bronk SF, Werneburg NW, Gores GJ. Free fatty acids induce JNK-dependent hepatocyte lipoapoptosis. The Journal of Biological Chemistry. 2006;**281**:12093-12101. DOI: 10.1074/jbc.M510660200

[100] Siler SQ, Neese RA, Hellerstein MK. De novo lipogenesis, lipid kinetics, and whole-body lipid balances in humans after acute alcohol consumption. The American Journal of Clinical Nutrition. 1999;**70**:928-936

[101] Boden G, She P, Mozzoli M, Cheung P, Gumireddy K, Reddy P, et al. Free fatty acids produce insulin resistance and activate the proinflammatory nuclear factor-kappaB pathway in rat liver. Diabetes. 2005;**54**:3458-3465

[102] Nicolas J, Fernández-Solà J. Increased circulating leptin levels in chronic alcoholism. Alcoholism, Clinical and Experimental Research. 2001;**25**(1):83-88

[103] Tang H, Sebastian BM, Axhemi A, Chen X, Hillian AD, Jacobsen DW, et al. Ethanol-induced oxidative stress via the CYP2E1 pathway disrupts adiponectin secretion from adipocytes. Alcoholism, Clinical and Experimental Research. 2012;**36**:214-222. DOI: 10.1111/j.1530-0277.2011.01607.x

[104] Xu J, Lai KKY, Verlinsky A, Lugea A, French SW, Cooper MP, et al. Synergistic steatohepatitis by moderate obesity and alcohol in mice despite increased adiponectin and p-AMPK. Journal of Hepatology. 2011;**55**:673-682. DOI: 10.1016/j.jhep.2010.12.034

[105] Czarnecki D, Rosińska Z, Żekanowska E, Ziółkowski M, Góralczyk B, Gorzelańczyk EJ, et al. Changes in concentration of visfatin during four weeks of inpatient treatment of alcohol dependent males. Alcoholism and Drug Addiction. 2015;**28**:173-181. DOI: 10.1016/j.alkona.2015.05.002

[106] Ren R-Z, Zhang X, Xu J, Zhang H-Q, Yu C-X, Cao M-F, et al. Chronic ethanol consumption increases the levels of chemerin in the serum and adipose tissue of humans and rats. Acta Pharmacologica Sinica. 2012;**33**:652-659. DOI: 10.1038/aps.2012.11

[107] Eisinger K, Krautbauer S, Wiest R, Weiss TS, Buechler C. Reduced serum chemerin in patients with more severe liver cirrhosis. Experimental and Molecular Pathology. 2015;**98**:208-213. DOI: 10.1016/j.yexmp.2015.01.010

[108] Ikejima K, Honda H, Yoshikawa M, Hirose M, Kitamura T, Takei Y, et al. Leptin augments inflammatory and profibrogenic responses in the murine liver induced by hepatotoxic chemicals. Hepatology. 2001;**34**:288-297. DOI: 10.1053/jhep.2001.26518

[109] Shen J, Sakaida I, Uchida K, Terai S, Okita K. Leptin enhances TNF-α production via p38 and JNK MAPK in LPS-stimulated Kupffer cells. Life Sciences. 2005;**77**:1502-1515. DOI: 10.1016/j.lfs.2005.04.004

[110] Voican CS, Njiké-Nakseu M, Boujedidi H, Barri-Ova N, Bouchet-Delbos L, Agostini H, et al. Alcohol withdrawal alleviates adipose tissue inflammation in patients with alcoholic liver disease. Liver

International. 2015;**35**:967-978. DOI: 10.1111/liv.12575

[111] Schwabe RF, Brenner DA. Mechanisms of liver injury. I. TNF-α-induced liver injury: Role of IKK, JNK, and ROS pathways. The American Journal of Physiology-Gastrointestinal and Liver Physiology. 2006;**290**:G583-G589. DOI: 10.1152/ajpgi.00422.2005

[112] Hong F, Radaeva S, Pan H, Tian Z, Veech R, Gao B. Interleukin 6 alleviates hepatic steatosis and ischemia/reperfusion injury in mice with fatty liver disease. Hepatology. 2004;**40**: 933-941. DOI: 10.1002/hep.20400

[113] Park EJ, Lee JH, Yu G-Y, He G, Ali SR, Holzer RG, et al. Dietary and genetic obesity promote liver inflammation and tumorigenesis by enhancing IL-6 and TNF expression. Cell. 2010;**140**:197-208. DOI: 10.1016/j.cell.2009.12.052

[114] Mandrekar P, Ambade A, Lim A, Szabo G, Catalano D. An essential role for monocyte chemoattractant protein-1 in alcoholic liver injury: Regulation of proinflammatory cytokines and hepatic steatosis in mice. Hepatology. 2011;**54**:2185-2197. DOI: 10.1002/hep.24599

[115] Nio Y, Yamauchi T, Iwabu M, Okada-Iwabu M, Funata M, Yamaguchi M, et al. Monocyte chemoattractant protein-1 (MCP-1) deficiency enhances alternatively activated M2 macrophages and ameliorates insulin resistance and fatty liver in lipoatrophic diabetic A-ZIP transgenic mice. Diabetologia. 2012;**55**:3350-3358. DOI: 10.1007/s00125-012-2710-2

[116] Koeck ES, Iordanskaia T, Sevilla S, Ferrante SC, Hubal MJ, Freishtat RJ, et al. Adipocyte exosomes induce transforming growth factor beta pathway dysregulation in hepatocytes: A novel paradigm for obesity-related liver disease. The Journal of Surgical Research. 2014;**192**:268-275. DOI: 10.1016/j.jss.2014.06.050

[117] Bala S, Csak T, Saha B, Zatsiorsky J, Kodys K, Catalano D, et al. The pro-inflammatory effects of miR-155 promote liver fibrosis and alcohol-induced steatohepatitis. Journal of Hepatology. 2016;**64**:1378-1387. DOI: 10.1016/j.jhep.2016.01.035

Section 3

Diseases Due to Disturbances in Adipose Tissue

Chapter 5

Adipose Tissue Inflammation and Metabolic Disorders

Felipe Henriques, Alexander H. Bedard and Miguel Luiz Batista Júnior

Abstract

Adipose tissue not only possesses an important role in the storage of excess nutrients but also acts as a critical immune and endocrine organ. Researchers and clinicians now consider adipose tissue to be an active endocrine organ that secretes various humoral factors called "adipokines," which imparts important systemic metabolic effects, from food intake to glucose tolerance. Along with its production of specialized adipokines, adipose tissue also secretes proinflammatory cytokines that likely contributes to the low-level systemic inflammation that has become a hallmark of various metabolic syndrome-associated chronic pathologies, such as obesity and cancer cachexia. These systemic effects may be mediated by communication networks arising from the multitude of resident adipose cells, including adipocytes, endothelial cells, neuronal cells, stem cells and other precursors, and a wide variety of immune cell populations that recent studies have demonstrated play a crucial role in the development of adipose inflammation and systemic metabolic abnormalities. In this chapter, we detail various molecular pathways linking excess adipose lipid storage to chronic inflammation and review the current knowledge as to what triggers obesity- and cachexia-associated inflammation in adipose tissue. Finally, we describe how the cross talk between adipose tissue inflammation and the non-adipocyte resident cells present in tissue is involved in this metabolic disruption.

Keywords: adipokines, remodeling, cross talk, cachexia, obesity

1. Introduction

In recent years, adipose tissue has rapidly emerged as a critical player in maintaining an organism's metabolic homeostasis through its canonical role in storing excess energy, as well as its emerging role in facilitating communication modalities critical to maintaining systemic metabolism. These diverse abilities possessed by adipose tissue directly results from its heterogeneous composition which allows for the integration and propagation of signals that influence whole-body homeostasis. To be effective in reacting to alterations within the organism, the adipose tissue must be dynamic and remodel itself in order to preserve the health of the organism. While remodeling allows for the maintenance of homeostasis, this mechanism may become compromised in certain metabolic diseases, such as cancer cachexia and obesity. Here, the influence of adipose heterogeneity on tissue remodeling in the context of cancer cachexia and obesity will be further discussed.

2. The adipose tissue

2.1 Adipose heterogeneity

Adipose tissue, or fat tissue, is classified in morphofunctional term into two distinct groups; (1) white adipose tissue (WAT), composed predominantly of unilocular adipocytes, with low mitochondrial density and low oxidative capacity, and (2) brown adipose tissue (BAT), predominantly composed of multilocular adipocytes, high mitochondrial density and oxidative capacity for the uptake and oxidation of fatty acids and glucose related to the maintenance and regulation of body temperature [1]. Other differences between the two types of adipose tissues are the depot localization, profile of secreted molecules, cell population, vascularization and also innervation [2–4]. While both of these adipose tissue groups contribute a significant role in maintaining systemic homeostasis, WAT is the primary site of metabolic dysregulation in many metabolic diseases [5, 6].

WAT is divided into two large depots, subcutaneous adipose tissue (scWAT) and visceral adipose tissue (vWAT). scWAT is present in the innermost layers of the skin (hypodermis), while vWAT is located in the internal organs [7]. In addition, it is well described, both in experimental and clinical research, that adipose tissue is a heterogeneous tissue, that presents different gene and protein expression profiles, as well as cellular composition depending on the location of the tissue [8, 9]. scWAT represents approximately 80% of the total fat mass in healthy individuals, while vWAT accounts for between 10 and 20% of the total body fat of lean men, and between 5 and 10% of total fat in women [10]. vWAT has been shown to be more metabolically responsive, and its accumulation has a higher correlation with obesity-related mortality [11].

The morphological composition of adipose tissue plays an important role in the homeostatic maintenance and tissue development. Adipose tissue is a special type of connective tissue composed of different cell types composed of approximately 50–70% adipocytes and 30–50% of stromal vascular fraction (SVF) cells, where the mesenchymal precursor cells, pre-adipocytes, fibroblasts, leukocytes, blood vessels, lymph nodes and nerves are present (**Figure 1**) [12–14]. Numerous studies have shown the cellular heterogeneity of adipose tissue is a critical component in the

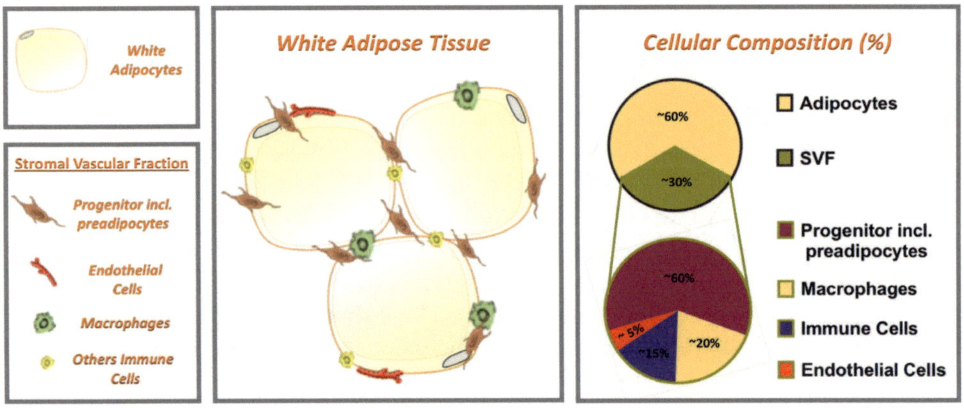

Figure 1.
Adipose tissue cellularity. The vast majority of the adipose tissue mass is composed of adipocytes (approximately 60%). There are many other cell types present in the adipose tissue. This specific portion of non-adipocytes is called the stromal vascular fraction (SVF) that is approximately 30% of the total cells in the tissue. In this portion are present mesenchymal precursor cells, pre-adipocytes, macrophages, others immune cells and endothelial cells.

tissue's ability to act as a hub of metabolic equilibrium [8, 15, 16]. Discovering and understanding the role of each cell present in adipose tissue leads to a greater chance in the development of possible therapeutics targeting metabolic disorders, which places a greater emphasis on studies of adipose cellularity.

2.2 Adipose tissue as an endocrine organ

This endocrine role of adipose tissue is best characterized by leptin [17, 18]. In 1994, with the discovery of leptin, the perception of WAT evolved from simply an energy storage compartment, mechanical protector and thermal insulation, but also an endocrine organ due the identification of a multitude of adipocyte-secreted factors that can act on distal tissues to regulate systemic functions, such as immunological and inflammatory responses, regulation of appetite, vascular events, control of reproductive functions, and insulin sensitivity [17, 19]. Total deficiency or insensitivity to leptin causes hyperphagia, morbid obesity, diabetes, a variety of neuroendocrine abnormalities, and autonomic and immunologic dysfunction [20].

Studies show that adipose tissue-derived hormones, fatty acids, lipids and signaling molecules, act by exerting endocrine, autocrine and paracrine effects. These factors are part of the large family of proteins and small molecules released by adipose tissue, which collectively are called adipokines [17, 21]. This tremendous diversity of signaling molecules enables the adipose tissue to engage in a wide array of signaling modalities that allows for systemic regulation of an organism's physiology (**Figure 2**). In instances of whole-body metabolic dysregulation, such as cancer cachexia and obesity, alterations to adipose tissue composition may have drastic effects on adipokine production. These effects are of critical importance in understanding the manifestation of metabolic syndromes. One example of such a dysregulation in adipokine profile is the release of pro- and anti- inflammatory adipokines during pathophysiological processes. This adipokine dysregulation

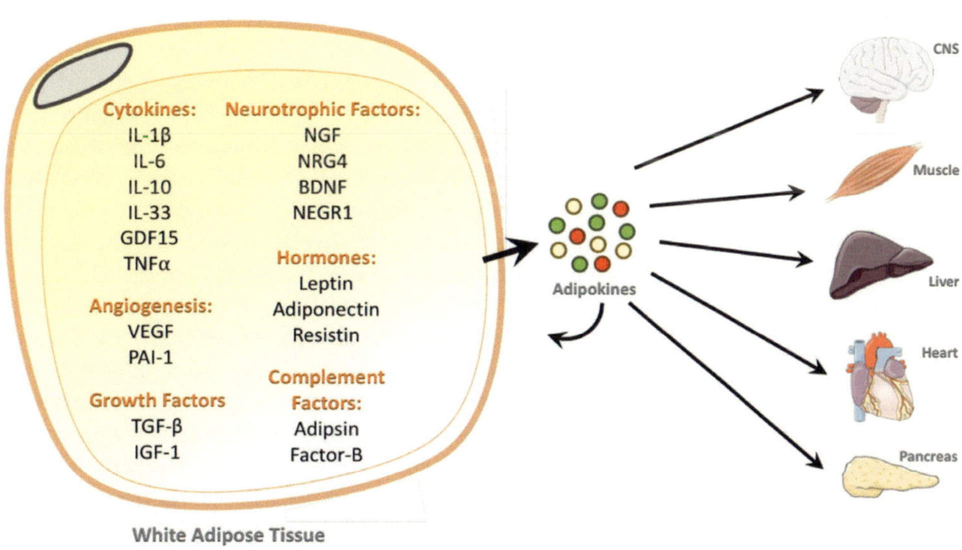

Figure 2.
Adipose tissue as endocrine organ. Endocrine factors released by white fat may signal to distant issues, including the brain, muscle, liver, heart and pancreas that regulate glucose and fatty acid metabolism in peripheral tissues, energy homeostasis, inflammatory response, and blood pressure, among others. Imbalanced secretion of some of these adipokines is associated with metabolic disorders. These factors released by white adipose tissue may target itself in an autocrine and paracrine manner, and also activate distant tissues in an endocrine manner (e.g., brown adipose tissue). Abbreviations see appendices and nomenclature section.

contributes significantly to the disruption of adipose tissue homeostasis in these diseases. Excessive secretion of potentially harmful adipokines (e.g., PAI-1, TNF-α and IL6) and hyposecretion of potentially beneficial adipokines, (e.g., adiponectin), may play an important role in the major mechanisms involved in during metabolic diseases. Thus, understanding the mechanism of various metabolic diseases calls for a deep understanding of the relationship between adipose tissue cellular composition and function.

2.3 Adipose tissue remodeling

Adipose tissue can respond rapidly and dynamically depending on the situation involved, thus fulfilling its major role in preserving whole-body energy homeostasis [22, 23]. Adipose tissue remodeling is a continuous process that is involved in some metabolic syndromes, such as reduction of vascular remodeling [24], overproduction of extracellular matrix [25], altered immune cell populations, and inflammatory responses are classic tissue response to such metabolic imbalances [26]. However, not all remodeling of adipose tissue is necessarily associated with pathological changes. A classic example is a concept of "metabolically healthy obesity" [27, 28], suggesting that some individuals may preserve systemic insulin sensitivity based on the "healthy" expansion of adipose tissue, avoiding the pathological consequences associated with obesity. Among the various consequences that can arise from adipose tissue remodeling is a state of local inflammation. This inflammatory state has been implicated in the progression of systemic dysregulation of metabolism in instances of "metabolically unhealthy obesity" [29]. Thus, comprehending the role of inflammation in the remodeling process of the adipose tissue is essential in understanding the main pathological alterations of this tissue.

2.3.1 An overview of adipose tissue inflammation

The adipose tissue plays host to a variety of immune cell populations that are intimately involved in the remodeling state of the tissue. Adipose tissue resident cells can secrete several proinflammatory cytokines that can orchestrate the inflammatory state of the tissue by influencing these immune cell populations within the tissue itself [21]. These inflammatory mediators have several metabolic and endocrine functions (immunity, metabolism, energy balance, among others), which is intimal related to the inflammatory process and immune system response [30, 31].

Inflammation in adipose tissue rose to prominence in the mid-1990s, shortly after obesity was recognized as an inflammatory disease in a study conducted with rats, which demonstrated greater expression of the gene encoding the pro-inflammatory cytokine TNF-α in adipose tissue, as well as a reduction in insulin sensitivity after exposure to a weight-gain diet [32]. In recent decades, data from human studies and transgenic animal models have strongly suggested correlative but also causative associations between the activation of proinflammatory pathways and insulin resistance [33, 34]. Particularly, chronic inflammation in adipose tissue appears to play an important role in the development of insulin resistance related to obesity and others metabolic diseases [33, 35]. The following potential mechanisms of adipose tissue inflammation and how this state is involved during the pathological process of cancer-associated cachexia and obesity are discussed.

2.3.2 Adipose tissue inflammation during cancer cachexia

Cancer cachexia syndrome is characterized by systemic inflammation, body weight loss, adipose tissue remodeling, and skeletal muscle wasting that cannot be fully reversed by conventional nutritional support and leads to progressive functional impairment [36]. Interesting, that adipose tissue of cachectic cancer patients is a possible relevant systemic source of inflammatory molecules during the development of the disease [37]. Moreover, it is now well described in both experimental and clinical research that these changes are dependent on the location of adipose tissue (e.g., visceral versus subcutaneous), which is involved in differential depot response to the disease [8, 38]. WAT also secretes and responds to pro-inflammatory mediators, as it also expresses several receptors for these secreted cytokines, chemokines, complement and growth factors [39]. These mediators act locally in an autocrine and/or paracrine manner, as well as distally in an endocrine fashion that can regulate appetite, modulate energy expenditure and affect a range of physiological processes, including insulin sensitivity and inflammatory responses [40].

Some interesting studies proposed that an imbalance between catabolic and anabolic processes in WAT is associated with the progression of cachexia. The proinflammatory cytokines interleukin 1-beta (IL-1β), interferon gamma (IFN-γ), interleukin 6 (IL-6) and tumor necrosis factor alpha (TNF-α) appear responsible for the activation of WAT catabolism in experimental models [37, 41–44]. Additionally, studies have demonstrated a predominance of an inflammatory profile in the terminal phase of the cachexia syndrome, notably within vWAT [45]. The presence of an important macrophage infiltration in this depot in rats with cancer cachexia was verified, which has been shown to contribute to the secretion of inflammatory factors [45]. More recently, in the same model of cancer cachexia, Batista et al. [41] showed an increase of macrophages around the adipocytes that were are polarized to a proinflammatory state in the vWAT simultaneously with the activation of the inflammasome pathway in this specific depot [43]. This event was immediately preceded by an increase in neutrophil density within the depot, which usually occurs in the intermediate phases of the syndrome. Therefore, depending on the inflammatory phase, distinct cell types can be observed. In fact, in several inflammatory processes, chronic inflammation is characterized by the presence of mononuclear cells that is usually preceded by tissue infiltration of neutrophils, which are cells that characterize acute inflammation [46].

In addition to animal models of cachexia, a study has recently demonstrated the presence of an exacerbated inflammatory profile in the WAT of humans with cancer cachexia [38]. In particular, an increase in CD68 positive cells, indicative of macrophages, and the clustering of the classic "crown-like structure" around the adipocyte were described. This morphological characteristic, although well-detailed in an obesity model, was described for the first time in cachexia. In the same study, an increase in CD3, a lymphocyte marker, and total collagen-positive cells in the WAT of these patients with cachexia was also detected. Taken together, the data indicate the presence of morphological alterations that suggest WAT remodeling in the presence of cachexia in humans [38].

However, despite the relevance of local inflammation, notably in WAT, the mechanisms that result in this process still require further detailing. Another important aspect is the characterization and understanding of the inflammatory process in this condition and its possible relation with the metabolic disorders, in order to answer if this process is secondary or the "trigger" for the development of the syndrome. Understanding the basic mechanisms of cancer cachexia that orchestrate WAT remodeling is relevant for the development of new pharmacological and nutritional therapies for anti-cachectic purposes. In this context, further demonstrating an intimate correlation between inflammation and the prognosis of cancer-associated cachexia, it was demonstrated that a genetic and pharmacological (atorvastatin) model of Toll-like receptor 4 (TLR4) inhibition, one of the primary inflammatory mediators, was able to attenuate classic symptoms of cachexia in an animal model [47]. This suggests that an important inflammatory pathway may be considered a promising target for therapeutic actions. It also further elucidates the mechanism by which cancer cachexia is manifested [47].

2.3.3 Adipose tissue inflammation during obesity

The incidence of overweight and obesity has increased substantially in the last decades worldwide is considered a worldwide epidemic, reducing the quality of life due to an increase in the physical and metabolic disability of individuals [48]. This occurs, at least partially, because of the obesity-induced insulin resistance and the fact that adipose tissue is not only an energy reservoir but also a secretory endocrine organ of cytokines, hormones, and proteins that affect the functionality of cells and tissues all over the body [49].

Recent studies have established association between obesity and systemic chronic low-grade inflammation [30, 50]. This association is characterized by, among other things, higher levels of circulating proinflammatory cytokines and fatty acids that can contribute to the development of the metabolic dysfunctions involved in the pathogenesis of its comorbidities [51].

It is well known that during this inflammation state in the adipose tissue, the tissue starts an intense remodeling in the adipose cell types present in the tissue. A major type of cell that plays an important role in the adipose tissue is the macrophages. Adipose tissue macrophage can be characterized in two different classes based on the expression of particular markers [52]. M1 macrophages or classically activated macrophages are characterized by *nitric oxide* synthase (*iNOS*) and CD11c surface expression, and expression of pro-inflammatory cytokines [53]. On the other hand, M2 macrophages or alternatively activated macrophages, are characterized by *Arginase* 1 (Arg1) and CD206 surface expression, and secrete anti-inflammatory cytokines predominates [53].

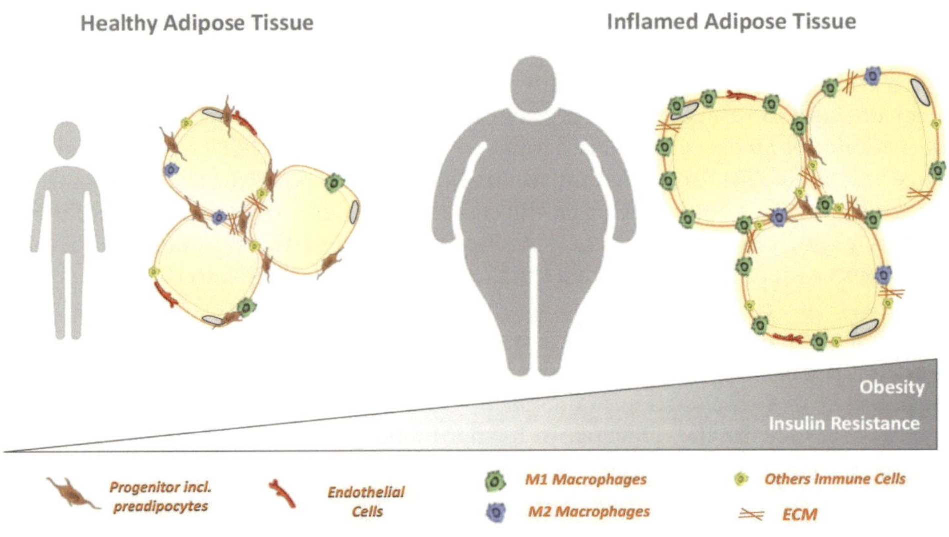

Figure 3.
Features in adipose tissue inflammation. Healthy adipose tissue displays high insulin sensitivity and is characterized by an anti-inflammatory state marked by elevated levels of adipocyte progenitor cells and M2 macrophages, sufficient vasculature to support tissue expansion and adipocyte hyperplasia. In an obese state, the adipose tissue contains hypertrophic adipocytes and a state of chronic inflammation exists within the tissue. A large increase in the populations of M1 proinflammatory macrophages, along with several other inflammatory leukocytes, begins to infiltrate the inflamed tissue. In addition, it is possible to observe a reduction in the vascularization of this unhealthy fat, resulting in a hypoxic state. Chronic inflammation results in the development of fibrotic structures in the form of increased extracellular components, such as collagen. Such events contribute to the development of insulin resistance.

A proposed model was defined as "phenotypic switching" that means an enhanced adipose tissue macrophage infiltration aggravates the environment of obesity-related inflammation [54]. This model emphasized that obesity starts to induced a polarization in these macrophage cells present in the tissue, that now the ratio M1/M2 macrophage are dysregulated and the M1 macrophage population are predominate in the adipose tissue [54]. Interesting that some studies showed that M1 macrophage population demonstrates a positive correlation with insulin resistance and an increase in proinflammatory responses [55]. Therefore, these studies suggest a sophisticated balance in relation to the diversity of macrophages population is necessary to sustain the adipose tissue homeostasis.

In addition to this deregulation in macrophages infiltration, other major changes also appear in the inflamed adipose tissue during obesity. Modifications in the composition of the extracellular matrix, decreased in the vascularization and alterations in the composition of immune cells in tissue are classic features of this adipose tissue remodeling [24, 26, 56] (**Figure 3**).

3. Concluding remarks

In summary, certain metabolic disease states, such as cancer cachexia and obesity, may alter the heterogeneous composition of adipose tissue, resulting in a remodeled tissue that is unable to properly respond to the systemic needs of the organism. We know that the adipose heterogeneity cells present in the tissue are the extremely importance in to regulate the homeostasis, and in the time that adipose tissue is affected to some metabolic syndrome this cross talk is deregulated and the homeostasis is compromised. After the adipose tissue is committed by a metabolic syndrome, the tissue starts to react in several ways. Several studies using cachexia and obesity experimental models have consistently indicated that a classic response to this imbalance, showed an intense adipose tissue remodeling in which the tissue begins to present numerous alterations in the morphology and also genetic alterations where its function ends up being extremely compromised. Finally, a deeper understanding of the initial stimulus and also who are the main types of cells involved in adipose tissue remodeling is essential for understanding the basic mechanisms in which adipose tissue performs. Once we have managed to obtain the answers to these important issues, we will be able to advance and have the chance to achieve some possible therapeutic target to these severe metabolic diseases.

Acknowledgements

The authors gratefully acknowledge the commitment and support by American Diabetes Association (ADA)—Grant #1-19-PMF-035.

Conflict of interest

The authors declare no conflicts of interest.

Appendices and nomenclature

BAT	brown adipose tissue
BDNF	brain-derived neurotrophic factor

ECM	extracellular matrix
GDF15	growth differentiation factor 15
IGF-1	insulin-like growth factor 1
IL6	interleukin 6
IL1β	interleukin 1β
IL10	interleukin 10
IL33	interleukin 33
NEGR1	neuronal growth regulator 1
NGF	nerve growth factor
NRG4	neuregulin 4
PAI-1	plasminogen activator inhibitor-1
scWAT	subcutaneous adipose tissue
SVF	stromal vascular fraction
TGF-β	transforming growth factor β
TLR4	Toll-like receptor 4
TNFα	tumor necrosis factor α
UCP1	uncoupling protein 1
vWAT	visceral adipose tissue
VEGF	vascular endothelial growth factor
WAT	white adipose tissue

Author details

Felipe Henriques[1]*, Alexander H. Bedard[1] and Miguel Luiz Batista Júnior[2]

1 Program in Molecular Medicine, University of Massachusetts Medical School, Worcester, MA, USA

2 Laboratory of Adipose Tissue Biology, Integrated Group of Biotechnology, University of Mogi das Cruzes, Mogi das Cruzes, SP, Brazil

*Address all correspondence to: felipe.henriques@umassmed.edu

References

[1] Cinti S. The adipose organ: Morphological perspectives of adipose tissues. The Proceedings of the Nutrition Society. 2001;**60**(3):319-328

[2] Bartelt A et al. Brown adipose tissue activity controls triglyceride clearance. Nature Medicine. 2011;**17**(2):200-205

[3] Rosell M et al. Brown and white adipose tissues: Intrinsic differences in gene expression and response to cold exposure in mice. American Journal of Physiology. Endocrinology and Metabolism. 2014;**306**(8):E945-E964

[4] Vidal-Puig A. Adipose tissue expandability, lipotoxicity and the metabolic syndrome. Endocrinología y Nutrición. 2013;**60**(Suppl 1):39-43

[5] Ghaben AL, Scherer PE. Adipogenesis and metabolic health. Nature Reviews. Molecular Cell Biology. 2019;**20**(4):242-258

[6] Wang L et al. PAI-1 exacerbates white adipose tissue dysfunction and metabolic dysregulation in high fat diet-induced obesity. Frontiers in Pharmacology. 2018;**9**:1087

[7] Ibrahim MM. Subcutaneous and visceral adipose tissue: Structural and functional differences. Obesity Reviews. 2010;**11**(1):11-18

[8] Batista ML Jr et al. Heterogeneous time-dependent response of adipose tissue during the development of cancer cachexia. The Journal of Endocrinology. 2012;**215**(3):363-373

[9] Cinti S. The adipose organ at a glance. Disease Models & Mechanisms. 2012;**5**(5):588-594

[10] Kaminski DA, Randall TD. Adaptive immunity and adipose tissue biology. Trends in Immunology. 2010;**31**(10):384-390

[11] Lafontan M, Girard J. Impact of visceral adipose tissue on liver metabolism. Part I: Heterogeneity of adipose tissue and functional properties of visceral adipose tissue. Diabetes & Metabolism. 2008;**34**(4 Pt 1):317-327

[12] Gesta S, Tseng YH, Kahn CR. Developmental origin of fat: Tracking obesity to its source. Cell. 2007;**131**(2):242-256

[13] Hausman GJ, Barb CR, Dean RG. Gene expression profiling in developing pig adipose tissue: Non-secreted regulatory proteins. Animal. 2011;**5**(7):1071-1081

[14] Guilherme A et al. Molecular pathways linking adipose innervation to insulin action in obesity and diabetes mellitus. Nature Reviews. Endocrinology. 2019;**15**(4):207-225

[15] Lee YH et al. Metabolic heterogeneity of activated beige/brite adipocytes in inguinal adipose tissue. Scientific Reports. 2017;7:39794

[16] Schoettl T, Fischer IP, Ussar S. Heterogeneity of adipose tissue in development and metabolic function. The Journal of Experimental Biology. 2018;**221**:jeb162958

[17] Kershaw EE, Flier JS. Adipose tissue as an endocrine organ. The Journal of Clinical Endocrinology and Metabolism. 2004;**89**(6):2548-2556

[18] Zhang Y et al. Positional cloning of the mouse obese gene and its human homologue. Nature. 1994;**372**(6505):425-432

[19] Trayhurn P, Wood IS. Signalling role of adipose tissue: Adipokines and inflammation in obesity. Biochemical Society Transactions. 2005;**33**(Pt 5): 1078-1081

[20] Harris RB. Direct and indirect effects of leptin on adipocyte metabolism. Biochimica et Biophysica Acta. 2014;**1842**(3):414-423

[21] Fantuzzi G. Adipose tissue, adipokines, and inflammation. The Journal of Allergy and Clinical Immunology. 2005;**115**(5):911-919. quiz 920

[22] Trujillo ME, Scherer PE. Adipose tissue-derived factors: Impact on health and disease. Endocrine Reviews. 2006;**27**(7):762-778

[23] Wernstedt Asterholm I et al. Adipocyte inflammation is essential for healthy adipose tissue expansion and remodeling. Cell Metabolism. 2014;**20**(1):103-118

[24] Sun K, Kusminski CM, Scherer PE. Adipose tissue remodeling and obesity. The Journal of Clinical Investigation. 2011;**121**(6):2094-2101

[25] Lin, Chun TH, Kang L. Adipose extracellular matrix remodelling in obesity and insulin resistance. Biochemical Pharmacology. 2016;**119**:8-16

[26] Choe SS et al. Adipose tissue remodeling: Its role in energy metabolism and metabolic disorders. Frontiers in Endocrinology. 2016;**7**:30

[27] Jung CH, Lee WJ, Song KH. Metabolically healthy obesity: A friend or foe? The Korean Journal of Internal Medicine. 2017;**32**(4):611-621

[28] Mongraw-Chaffin M et al. Metabolically healthy obesity, transition to metabolic syndrome, and cardiovascular risk. Journal of the American College of Cardiology. 2018;**71**(17):1857-1865

[29] Iacobini C et al. Metabolically healthy versus metabolically unhealthy obesity. Metabolism. 2019;**92**:51-60

[30] Monteiro R, Azevedo I. Chronic inflammation in obesity and the metabolic syndrome. Mediators of Inflammation. 2010;**2010**(289645):1-10

[31] Sharma P. Inflammation and the metabolic syndrome. Indian Journal of Clinical Biochemistry. 2011;**26**(4):317-318

[32] Hotamisligil GS, Shargill NS, Spiegelman BM. Adipose expression of tumor necrosis factor-alpha: Direct role in obesity-linked insulin resistance. Science. 1993;**259**(5091):87-91

[33] de Luca C, Olefsky JM. Inflammation and insulin resistance. FEBS Letters. 2008;**582**(1):97-105

[34] Shoelson SE, Lee J, Goldfine AB. Inflammation and insulin resistance. The Journal of Clinical Investigation. 2006;**116**(7):1793-1801

[35] Czech MP. Insulin action and resistance in obesity and type 2 diabetes. Nature Medicine. 2017;**23**(7):804-814

[36] Fearon K, Arends J, Baracos V. Understanding the mechanisms and treatment options in cancer cachexia. Nature Reviews. Clinical Oncology. 2013;**10**(2):90-99

[37] Batista ML Jr et al. Adipose tissue-derived factors as potential biomarkers in cachectic cancer patients. Cytokine. 2013;**61**(2):532-539

[38] Batista ML Jr et al. Cachexia-associated adipose tissue morphological rearrangement in gastrointestinal cancer patients. Journal of Cachexia, Sarcopenia and Muscle. 2016;**7**(1):37-47

[39] Arner P. The adipocyte in insulin resistance: Key molecules and the impact of the thiazolidinediones. Trends in Endocrinology and Metabolism. 2003;**14**(3):137-145

[40] Mantovani A et al. Cancer-related inflammation. Nature. 2008;**454**(7203):436-444

[41] Batista ML Jr et al. Adipose tissue inflammation and cancer cachexia: Possible role of nuclear transcription factors. Cytokine. 2012;**57**(1):9-16

[42] Beluzi M et al. Pioglitazone treatment increases survival and prevents body weight loss in tumor-bearing animals: Possible anti-cachectic effect. PLoS One. 2015;**10**(3):e0122660

[43] Neves RX et al. White adipose tissue cells and the progression of cachexia: Inflammatory pathways. Journal of Cachexia, Sarcopenia and Muscle. 2016;**7**(2):193-203

[44] Lopes MA et al. LLC tumor cells-derivated factors reduces adipogenesis in co-culture system. Heliyon. 2018;**4**(7):e00708

[45] Machado AP, Costa Rosa LF, Seelaender MC. Adipose tissue in Walker 256 tumour-induced cachexia: Possible association between decreased leptin concentration and mononuclear cell infiltration. Cell and Tissue Research. 2004;**318**(3):503-514

[46] Schymeinsky J, Mocsai A, Walzog B. Neutrophil activation via beta2 integrins (CD11/CD18): Molecular mechanisms and clinical implications. Thrombosis and Haemostasis. 2007;**98**(2):262-273

[47] Henriques F et al. Toll-like receptor-4 disruption suppresses adipose tissue remodeling and increases survival in cancer cachexia syndrome. Scientific Reports. 2018;**8**(1):18024

[48] Ng M et al. Global, regional, and national prevalence of overweight and obesity in children and adults during 1980-2013: A systematic analysis for the global burden of disease study. Lancet. 2013;**2014, 384**(9945):766-781

[49] Coelho M, Oliveira T, Fernandes R. Biochemistry of adipose tissue: An endocrine organ. Archives of Medical Science. 2013;**9**(2):191-200

[50] Pereira SS, Alvarez-Leite JI. Low-grade inflammation, obesity, and diabetes. Current Obesity Reports. 2014;**3**(4):422-431

[51] Rehman K, Akash MS. Mechanisms of inflammatory responses and development of insulin resistance: How are they interlinked? Journal of Biomedical Science. 2016;**23**(1):87

[52] Chylikova J et al. M1/M2 macrophage polarization in human obese adipose tissue. Biomedical Papers of the Medical Faculty of the University Palacky, Olomouc, Czech Republic. 2018;**162**(2):79-82

[53] Weisser SB et al. Generation and characterization of murine alternatively activated macrophages. Methods in Molecular Biology. 2013;**946**:225-239

[54] Lumeng CN et al. Phenotypic switching of adipose tissue macrophages with obesity is generated by spatiotemporal differences in macrophage subtypes. Diabetes. 2008;**57**(12):3239-3246

[55] Castoldi A et al. The macrophage switch in obesity development. Frontiers in Immunology. 2015;**6**:637

[56] Strissel KJ et al. Adipocyte death, adipose tissue remodeling, and obesity complications. Diabetes. 2007;**56**(12):2910-2918

Chapter 6

Lipedema: A Painful Adipose Tissue Disorder

Sara Al-Ghadban, Karen L. Herbst and Bruce A. Bunnell

Abstract

Lipedema is a painful fat disease of loose connective tissue usually misdiagnosed as lifestyle-induced obesity that affects ~10% of women of European descent as well as other populations. Lipedema is characterized by symmetric enlargement of the buttocks, hips, and legs due to increased loose connective tissue; arms are also affected in 80% of patients. Lipedema loose connective tissue is characterized by hypertrophic adipocytes, inflammatory cells, and dilated leaky blood and lymphatic vessels. Altered fluid flux through the tissue causes accumulation of fluid, protein, and other constituents in the interstitium resulting in recruitment of inflammatory cells, which in turn stimulates fibrosis and results in difficulty in weight loss. Inflammation and excess interstitial substance may also activate nerve fibers instigating the painful lipedema fat tissue. More research is needed to characterize lipedema loose connective tissue structure in depth, as well as the form and function of blood and lymphatic vessels. Understanding the pathophysiology of the disease will allow healthcare providers to diagnose the disease and develop treatments.

Keywords: lipedema, symptoms, diagnosis, treatment, blood vessels, lymphatics

1. Introduction

Loose connective tissue disorders include lipedema, Dercum's disease (DD), familial multiple lipomatosis (FML) and multiple symmetric lipomatosis (MSL). All these disorders share many similarities with lipedema including painful lipomas, obesity, fibrosis, a risk of developing lymphedema and difficulty in losing the abnormal fat through diet and exercise. There are clinical characteristics specific for lipedema, including the onset of the disease, fat location and associated health issues (**Table 1**) [1, 2].

Lipedema is often misdiagnosed as lifestyle-induced obesity that affects ~10% of women of European descent as well as other populations [3, 4]. Although both disorders are considered inflammatory diseases due to the presence of increased macrophages and hypertrophic adipocytes, there are significant differences between the two disorders. Among these is the location of the fat, primarily abdominal or spread widely over the body in obesity compared to the symmetric distribution in the lower extremities in lipedema, the texture of the skin (thin and soft in lipedema and thicker in obesity), easy bruising and pain upon the introduction of pressure in lipedema [5, 6].

Characteristic	Lipedema	DD	MSL	FML	MSL
Abnormal fat location	Legs, arms, abdomen	Global	Upper; can be global	Arms, thighs, trunk, abdomen	Upper; can be global
Diet-resistant fat	Yes	Yes	Yes	Yes	Yes
Lipomas	Yes	Common	Common in men	Common	Common in men
Time fat change	Puberty; 3rd decade	Child-adult	Adult; child rare	Child-adult	Adult; child rare
Painful fat	Yes	Yes	Not usually	Lipoma	Not usually
Sex predominance	Female	Female	Male	Male = female	Male
Lymphatic dysfunction	Yes	Yes	Yes	Yes	Yes
Prevalence	Possibly common	Possibly common	Rare	Rare	Rare
Associated conditions	Lymphedema	Autoimmune; diabetes	Neuropathy	Moles; neuropathy	Neuropathy
Inheritance pattern	Autosomal dominant; incomplete penetrance	Autosomal dominant; sex-specific influence	Autosomal dominant or recessive	Autosomal dominant	Autosomal dominant or recessive

Modified from Ref. [1].

Table 1.
Characteristics of loose connective tissue disorders.

The focus of this review will be on the disease of lipedema, different stages and types, diagnosis and treatment, pathogenesis and current research in the field.

2. Lipedema

Lipedema also referred to as lipedema, is a painful loose connective tissue disorder first described in 1940 by Allen and Hines [7]. Lipedema is characterized by symmetric enlargement of the buttocks, hips and legs due to deposition of loose connective tissue that includes fascia, adipocytes, immune cells and other structures; arms are also affected in 80% of patients [3, 4]. Feet are typically spared, but ankle cuffs are often noted in advanced stages of lipedema where the risk of lymphedema is also high [8, 9]. Patients with lipedema experience mobility issues, psychosocial distress, anxiety, eating disorders, sleep apnea and depression [1, 10].

Lipedema is considered a hormone-related disorder affecting almost exclusively women during puberty, childbirth or menopause. Case reports of men with lipedema have been described in literature. Men with lipedema have elevated estrogen level and low to absent testosterone levels resulting in cirrhosis, gynecomastia and hypogonadism [11–13]. While the exact etiopathogenesis of this disease is unknown [10, 14], many studies have demonstrated that inflammatory cells, hypertrophic adipocytes, abnormal blood vessels and lymphatic dysfunction are associated with tissue damage and development of a fibrotic disease [14–17].

2.1 Stages of lipedema

Lipedema consists of three stages characterized by the texture of skin and tissue formation. Stage 1 involves smooth skin over pearl-sized nodules in a hypertrophic fat layer; Stage 2 has skin indentations over a hypertrophic fat structure of pearl-to-apple-size masses; and Stage 3 includes pearl-sized nodules and much larger fat masses causing lobules of skin and fat to form mainly on the hips, thighs, and around the knees. Lymphedema, causing fluid accumulation in the limbs, may develop during any stage of lipedema and is referred to as lipo-lymphedema [1, 3, 10, 18, 19].

Healthcare providers often misdiagnose women with lipedema as they do not take into account the disproportionate size of the legs compared to trunk especially in Stage 1 and 2 along with the inability to lose fat from areas affected by lipedema. It is possible to confuse women with Stage 3 lipedema as having lifestyle-induced obesity due to fat involving more areas of the body.

2.2 Types of lipedema

In addition to stages of lipedema, lipedema is also characterized by types determined by the area of the body that is affected. There are five types of lipedema; types I, II, and III are the most common. In Type I, fat is deposited in the areas of the buttocks and hips resembling saddle bags. In Type II, fat extends to the knees from the buttocks area with the formation of folds of fat around the inside of the knee. In Type III, fat spreads all over the lower body from the hips to the ankles. In Type IV, upper arms are affected causing difficulty in lifting the arm and stress on the shoulder. In Type V, fat is restricted to the lower legs. It is worth noting that patients with lipedema can clinically present with a mixture of types [3, 10].

2.3 Signs and symptoms

Pain, tenderness, bruising easily, symmetrical swelling of the legs, heaviness of affected limbs, burning sensations in the skin and fat, soft skin, negative stemmer's sign and hypermobile joints are among the common symptoms observed in lipedema patients [2, 3, 6, 13]. Hypermobility in women with has been reported to contribute to joint damage and increase the risk of cardiovascular disease as seen in Ehlers Danlos Syndrome-Hypermobility Type (EDS-HT) with Beighton score higher than 5 [2, 3, 20, 21]. Thus, hypermobility causes structural changes in lipedema tissue resulting in increased fibrosis, dysfunction of blood vessels and accumulation of interstitial fluid.

Women with lipedema also experience emotional symptoms due to unexplained weight gain including embarrassment, anxiety and depression that impact their overall quality of life [22, 23]. Symptoms may progress in advanced stages of lipedema that might be associated with increased cardiovascular and renal diseases. A study conducted by Herbst el al. in 2015 provides a detailed list of symptoms experienced by lipedema patients [3].

2.4 Diagnosis and treatment of lipedema

Diagnosis of lipedema involves a comprehensive physical exam based on the criteria listed by Wold and colleagues in 1951, [4] medical and surgical history, list of medications that might affect weight or fluid retention and family history. A physical examination includes assessment of the enlarged lower extremities carefully noting the texture of the affected areas such as velvety soft skin that can be found in hypermobility, nodular fat, pain when applying pressure, tenderness upon palpation and accumulation of fluid such as pitting or non-pitting edema which may indicate lymphedema [18, 24]. Bruising caused by increased capillary fragility [6], spider veins and telangiectasia showing on the surface of the skin due to venous insufficiency are also observed in lipedema patients [4, 10].

Although, there is no cure for lipedema, treatments like liposuction (tumescent and water jet) [25], complete decongestive therapy that includes manual lymphatic drainage [26, 27], compression garments, a healthy diet, physical activity, medications and supplements (statins, selenium, diosmin, amphetamines and butcher's broom) have been shown to reduce pain, improve lymphatic function, decrease leakage from blood vessels, lessen inflammation and fibrosis and maintain a healthy gut [24, 28–34].

Liposuction is by far the most effective treatment to decrease the fibrotic lipedema fat and thereby maintain mobility which is essential for the welfare of women living with lipedema [35–37]. Water jet-assisted liposuction has been proven to be as effective as tumescent liposuction. Damage to the lymph vessels has not been show as evidenced in a histological study conducted by Stutz et al. on lipoaspirates collected from lipedema patients [32]. Nevertheless, special care should be taken with lipo-lymphedema patients, where accumulated lymph and or fibrotic tissue should be removed first. Furthermore, follow-up and compression therapy are advised for successful and effective treatment.

Deep tissue massage has also been demonstrated to improve the quality of subcutaneous adipose tissue by decreasing pain, fibrosis and fat tissue in women with lipedema [29, 38].

Additionally, a healthy non-inflammatory diet is highly recommended, even though it will not reduce the lipedema tissue, but it might slow the progression of the disease by reducing inflammation and pain, lessen the swelling and ultimately improve quality of life. No one plan works for everyone but a ketogenic diet with low processed carbohydrate and mild physical exercises like walking, swimming, Pilates, yoga and other home excise programs are suggested by lipedema specialists. These activates will help the function of lymphatic pump and maintain a normal metabolism.

Finally, it is very important to detect and treat lipedema at early stages thus preventing the complications that might occur due to the progression of disease. These complications comprise eating disorders, sleep apnea, diabetes mellitus, arthritis, hypertension, cellulitis, cardiac and renal disease.

3. Lipedema versus lymphedema

There are distinctive criteria for lipedema which are absent in lymphedema including a negative Stemmer's sign, minimal pitting edema, thin skin, easy bruising, tenderness and pain [14, 39, 40]. Although lymphatic microaneurysms might develop in the later stages of lipedema leading to secondary lymphedema, imaging techniques like high-resolution cutaneous ultrasonography and magnetic resonance imaging showed no defects in the lymphatic system in early stages [24, 41–43]. Other methods have also been successfully used to differentiate lipedema from lymphedema which includes tissue dielectric constant and dual-energy X-ray absorptiometry techniques [44–48].

Dysfunction of lymphatic vessels results in accumulation of interstitial fluid (edema) in adipose tissues triggering inflammation by the recruitment of macrophages resulting in fibrosis and difficulty with weight loss. As a consequence, adipose tissue loses its elasticity suggesting that lipedema might be a connective tissue disorder [15, 49]. Studies have also indicated that edema might induce growth of lipedema fat as well as hypoxia resulting in adipocyte cell death [50].

Further, morphologic changes in lymphatic vessels and accumulation of interstitial fluid are present in some women with lipedema, with no change in transport of lymphatic fluid, which suggests these individuals might have a higher risk of progressing to lipo-lymphedema especially in advanced stages of lipedema [15, 51]. Accurate diagnosis of lipedema in association with lymphedema is essential for treating and following up of lipedema patients.

4. Pathophysiology of the disease

Hormones, genetic factors, leaky blood vessels, dysfunctional lymphatics system, inflammation, hypertrophic adipocytes and interstitial thickening are among the factors that contribute to the pathogenesis of lipedema [10, 12, 15].

4.1 Hormones

Hormones play an essential role in the etiology of the lipedema, but how they affect the metabolism and function of adipocytes function is still unknown. Studies have shown that hormones, like estrogen and progesterone, have a direct effect on lipogenesis, insulin levels and adipose tissue distribution in the body. Dysregulation of hormonal levels lead to fat dysregulation, impairment of the lipogenesis-lipolysis mechanism, hypertension, insulin resistance and hyperinsulinemia [13, 52, 53]. Hormones might also have an impact on the nervous system which might explain the pain experienced by lipedema patients. Szél et al. hypothesized that alteration in estrogen (or estrogen receptors) maybe involved in the pathogenesis of lipedema by suggesting a link between accumulation of adipose tissue, imbalanced estrogen levels and inflammation of the peripheral and sympathetic nerves of the disease [13].

4.2 Adipocytes, immune cells and blood vessels

Lipedema fat tissue is characterized by hypertrophic adipocytes, inflammatory immune cells, dilation of subdermal blood and lymphatic vessels. We and others have shown a high number of infiltrating macrophages in lipedema adipose tissue detected by the CD68 marker and observed as around blood vessels or as crown-like structures surrounding necrotic adipocytes. In addition to macrophages, mast cells and T-lymphocytes were detected in hyper-vascular areas mainly around blood vessels in lipedema fat tissue which might contribute to capillary permeability and accumulation of interstitial fluid [15, 16, 54].

An article published in 2004 by Taylor et al. showed that accumulation of mast cells in lipedema tissue contributed to increased interstitial fluid, deterioration of adipocytes and potentially elastic fiber fragmentation due to the release of elastase [55], confirming that lipedema is a connective tissue disorder. Adding to that, direct cell-cell interaction between hypertrophic adipocyte and macrophages as well as secreted paracrine factors such as vascular endothelial growth factor (VEGF), a marker of angiogenesis, previously reported in the blood of women with lipedema [56] might be associated with increase in the number of blood vessels, dilation of capillaries, hypoxia, inflammation and tissue fibrosis found in lipedema patients [15, 18, 57].

5. Is there a role of adipose-derived stem cells (ASC) in lipedema?

Adipose tissue-derived stem cells are widely studied for their immunomodulatory, anti-inflammatory, anti-fibrotic, anti-apoptotic and pro-angiogenic effects

[58–60], but how ASCs contribute to the development of lipedema has not been investigated yet. Due to their high therapeutic potential, ASCs are now considered an indispensable tool in regenerative medicine [61–64]. Studies have shown the successful treatment with ASCs for many disease including graft-versus-host disease [65], wound healing [66], cardiovascular [67], inflammatory bowel disease [68], diabetes mellitus [69] and several injuries including kidney and spinal cord [70], bone and craniofacial reconstruction [71, 72], liver cirrhosis [73], multiple sclerosis [74]. In addition to their self-renewal ability, ASCs have the ability to differentiate into multiple lineages, including adipocytes, osteoblasts, chondrocytes, and endothelial cells [75, 76]. Thus, ASCs might play a role in lipedema adiposity by inducing the expansion and differentiation of progenitor adipose-derived stem/progenitor cells (pre-adipocytes) into mature adipocytes (hyperplasia). Suga el at. have shown an increase in proliferation of adipose-derived stem/progenitor cell proliferation using Ki67 and CD34 markers suggesting an increase in adipogenesis, hypoxia, and adipocyte necrosis, at least in one case [16].

Adding to that, inflammatory cytokines secreted by hypertrophic adipocytes and factors in the interstitial fluid could stimulate ASC differentiation into mature adipocytes. Alternatively, ASCs produce a plethora of pro- and anti-inflammatory cytokines that might contribute to angiogenesis and inflammation resulting in leaky and fragile blood vessels [77, 78]. Priglinger et al. have characterized lipedema ASCs isolated from liposuction samples and showed an increasing number of endothelial/pericytic cells using CD146 marker in lipedema patients compared to healthy individuals proposing that this increase might be a marker of repair of leaky blood and lymphatic vessels in lipedema tissues [54].

Although, ASCs might induce adipogenesis in lipedema an in-depth characterization of ASCs is required to confirm this theory. Otherwise, if ASCs prove to have anti-inflammatory, anti-fibrotic or pro-angiogenic effects, then they might be used to lessen tissue damage caused by leaky vessels; hence autologous treatment might be a promising tool for lipedema patients.

6. Conclusion

Lipedema is a painful fat disease that should be differentiated from obesity and lymphedema. It is the responsibility of the healthcare provider to determine the accurate diagnosis of the disease for successful treatment and management. Liposuction, hands-on therapy, exercise, and a healthy eating plan are recommended for lipedema patients. Although the etiology of lipedema is complicated, hypertrophic adipocytes, inflammatory cytokines, and macrophages, hypoxia, leaky vessels and accumulation of interstitial fluid contribute to the pathogenesis of the disease and may also help guide treatment.

Acknowledgements

This work was funded by a grant from the Lipedema Foundation.

Conflict of interest

The authors declare no conflict of interest.

DOI: http://dx.doi.org/10.5772/intechopen.88632

Author details

Sara Al-Ghadban[1*], Karen L. Herbst[2] and Bruce A. Bunnell[1,3]

1 Center for Stem Cell Research and Regenerative Medicine, Tulane University School of Medicine, New Orleans, LA, USA

2 Department of Medicine and TREAT Program, College of Medicine, University of Arizona, Tucson, Arizona, USA

3 Department of Pharmacology, School of Medicine, Tulane University, New Orleans, LA, USA

*Address all correspondence to: sara.ghadban@gmail.com

References

[1] Herbst KL. Rare adipose disorders (RADs) masquerading as obesity. Acta Pharmacologica Sinica. 2012;**33**(2):155-172

[2] Beltran K, Herbst KL. Differentiating lipedema and Dercum's disease. International Journal of Obesity. 2017;**41**(2):240-245

[3] Herbst KL et al. Lipedema fat and signs and symptoms of illness, increase with advancing stage. Archives of Medicine. 2015;**7**:1-8

[4] Wold LE, Hines EA, Allen EV. Lipedema of the legs; a syndrome characterized by fat legs and edema. Annals of Internal Medicine. 1951;**34**(5):1243

[5] Forner-Cordero I et al. Lipedema: An overview of its clinical manifestations, diagnosis and treatment of the disproportional fatty deposition syndrome—Systematic review. Clinical Obesity. 2012;**2**(3-4):86-95

[6] Szolnoky G et al. Measurement of capillary fragility: A useful tool to differentiate lipedema from obesity? Lymphology. 2017;**50**(4):203

[7] Wold LE, Hines EA, Allen EA. Lipedema of the legs: A syndrome characterised by fat legs and orthostatic edema. Proceedings of the Staff Meetings. Mayo Clinic. 1940;**15**:184-187

[8] Shin BW et al. Lipedema, a rare disease. Annals of Rehabilitation Medicine. 2011;**35**(6):922

[9] Szolnoky G, Kemeny L. Lipoedema: From clinical presentation to therapy. Further aspects. The British Journal of Dermatology. 2010;**162**(4):889-889

[10] Torre YS-DL et al. Lipedema: Friend and foe. Hormone Molecular Biology and Clinical Investigation. 2018;**33**(1). DOI: 10.1515/hmbci-2017-0076

[11] Chen S-G et al. Painful fat syndrome in a male patient. British Journal of Plastic Surgery. 2004;**57**(3):282-286

[12] Child AH et al. Lipedema: An inherited condition. American Journal of Medical Genetics Part A. 2010;**152**(4):970-976

[13] Szél E et al. Pathophysiological dilemmas of lipedema. Medical Hypotheses. 2014;**83**(5):599-606

[14] Buck DW, Herbst KL. Lipedema: A relatively common disease with extremely common misconceptions. Plastic and Reconstructive Surgery. Global Open. 2016;**4**(9):e1043

[15] Al-Ghadban S et al. Dilated blood and lymphatic microvessels, angiogenesis, increased macrophages, and adipocyte hypertrophy in lipedema thigh skin and fat tissue. Journal of Obesity. 2019;**2019**:8747461

[16] Suga H et al. Adipose tissue remodeling in lipedema: Adipocyte death and concurrent regeneration. Journal of Cutaneous Pathology. 2009;**36**(12):1293-1298

[17] Lohrmann C, Foeldi E, Langer M. MR imaging of the lymphatic system in patients with lipedema and lipo-lymphedema. Microvascular Research. 2009;**77**(3):335-339

[18] Fife EC, Maus AE, Carter JM. Lipedema: A frequently misdiagnosed and misunderstood fatty deposition syndrome. Advances in Skin & Wound Care. 2010;**23**(2):81-92

[19] Pascucci A, Lynch PJ. Lipedema with multiple lipomas. Dermatology Online Journal. 2010;**16**(9):4

[20] Strunk RG, Pfefer MT, Dube D. Multimodal chiropractic care of pain and disability for a patient diagnosed with benign joint hypermobility syndrome: A case report. Journal of Chiropractic Medicine. 2014;**13**(1):35-42

[21] Beighton P, Grahame R, Bird H. Assessment of Hypermobility. London: Springer London; 2012. pp. 11-26

[22] Alwardat N et al. The effect of lipedema on health-related quality of life and psychological status: A narrative review of the literature. Eat Weight Disorder. 2019. https://doi.org/10.1007/s40519-019-00703-x

[23] Dudek JE et al. Depression and appearance-related distress in functioning with lipedema. Psychology. Health & Medicine. 2018;**23**(7):846-853

[24] Peled AW, Kappos EA. Lipedema: Diagnostic and management challenges. International Journal of Women's Health. 2016;**8**:389

[25] Schmeller W, Hueppe M, Meier-Vollrath I. Tumescent liposuction in lipoedema yields good long-term results. British Journal of Dermatology. 2012;**166**(1):161-168

[26] Szolnoky G et al. Complete decongestive physiotherapy with and without pneumatic compression for treatment of lipedema: A pilot study. Lymphology. 2008;**41**(1):40

[27] Szolnoky G et al. Complex decongestive physiotherapy decreases capillary fragility in lipedema. Lymphology. 2008;**41**(4):161

[28] Okhovat J-P, Alavi A. In: Rerkasem K, editor. Lipedema: A Review of the Literature. Los Angeles, CA: SAGE Journals; 2015. pp. 262-267

[29] Herbst KL, Ussery C, Eekema A. Pilot study: Whole body manual subcutaneous adipose tissue (SAT) therapy improved pain and SAT structure in women with lipedema. Hormone Molecular Biology and Clinical Investigation. 2017;**33**(2). DOI: 10.1515/hmbci-2017-0035

[30] Chuck Ehrlich EI, Herbst KL, Kahn L-A, Sears DD, Kenyon M, McMahon E. Lymphedema and Lipedema Nutrition Guide. Foods, Vitamins, Minerals, and Supplements. San Francisco: Lymph Notes; 2015

[31] Beninson J, Edelglass JW. Lipedema—The non-lymphatic masquerader. Angiology. 1984;**35**(8):506

[32] Stutz J, Krahl D. Water jet-assisted liposuction for patients with lipoedema: Histologic and immunohistologic analysis of the aspirates of 30 lipoedema patients. Aesthetic Plastic Surgery. 2009;**33**(2):153-162

[33] Portillo-Soto A et al. Comparison of blood flow changes with soft tissue mobilization and massage therapy. Journal of Alternative and Complementary Medicine (New York, N.Y.). 2014;**20**(12):932

[34] Macdonald JM, Sims N, Mayrovitz HN. Lymphedema, lipedema, and the open wound: The role of compression therapy. Surgical Clinics of North America. 2003;**83**(3):639-658

[35] Dadras M et al. Liposuction in the treatment of lipedema: A longitudinal study. Archives of Plastic Surgery. 2017;**44**(4):324-331

[36] Brorson H. Liposuction normalizes—In contrast to other therapies—Lymphedema-induced adipose tissue hypertrophy. Handchirurgie, Mikrochirurgie, Plastische Chirurgie. 2013;**44**(06):348-354

[37] Baum S et al. Treatment of lipoedema using liposuction: Results

of our own surveys. Phlébologie. 2015;**44**(3):121-132

[38] Ibarra M et al. Subcutaneous adipose tissue therapy reduces fat by dual X-ray absorptiometry scan and improves tissue structure by ultrasound in women with lipoedema and Dercum disease. Clinical Obesity. 2018;**8**(6):398-406

[39] Shavit E, Wollina U, Alavi A. Lipoedema is not lymphoedema: A review of current literature. International Wound Journal. 2018;**15**(6):921-928

[40] Rudkin G, Miller TA. Lipedema—A clinical entity distinct from lymphedema. Plastic and Reconstructive Surgery. 1994;**94**(6):841-847

[41] Langendoen SI et al. Lipoedema: From clinical presentation to therapy. A review of the literature. British Journal of Dermatology. 2009;**161**:980-986

[42] Fonder MA, Loveless JW, Lazarus G. Lipedema, a frequently unrecognized problem. Journal of the American Academy of Dermatology. 2007;**57**(2):S1-S3

[43] Amann-Vesti B, Franzeck UK, Bollinger A. Microlymphatic aneurysms in patients with lipedema. Lymphology. 2001;**34**(4):170-175

[44] Dimakakos PB et al. MRI and ultrasonographic findings in the investigation of lymphedema and lipedema. International Surgery. 1997;**82**(4):411

[45] Naouri M et al. High-resolution cutaneous ultrasonography to differentiate lipoedema from lymphoedema. British Journal of Dermatology. 2010;**163**(2):296-301

[46] Bräutigam P et al. Analysis of lymphatic drainage in various forms of leg edema using two compartment lymphoscintigraphy. Lymphology. 1998;**31**(2):43

[47] Tuğral A, Bakar Y. An approach to lipedema: A literature review of current knowledge of an underestimated health problem. European Journal of Plastic Surgery. 2019. https://doi.org/10.1007/s00238-019-01519-9

[48] Birkballe S. Can tissue dielectric constant measurement aid in differentiating lymphoedema from lipoedema in women with swollen legs? British Journal of Dermatology. 2014;**170**(1):96-103

[49] Williams A, Macewan I. Accurate diagnosis and self-care support for women with lipoedema. Practice Nursing. 2016;**27**(7):325-332

[50] Martin S, Edward MC, Peter C. Lymph makes you fat. Nature Genetics. 2005;**37**(10):1023

[51] Bilancini S et al. Functional lymphatic alterations in patients suffering from lipedema. Angiology. 1995;**46**(4):333-339

[52] Van Pelt R et al. Acute modulation of adipose tissue lipolysis by intravenous estrogens. Obesity. 2006;**14**(12):2163-2172

[53] Mayes JS, Watson GH. Direct effects of sex steroid hormones on adipose tissues and obesity. Obesity Reviews. 2004;**5**(4):197-216

[54] Priglinger E et al. The adipose tissue: Derived stromal vascular fraction cells from lipedema patients: Are they different? Cytotherapy. 2017;**19**(7):849-860

[55] Taylor NE et al. Tumefactive lipedema with pseudoxanthoma elasticum-like microscopic changes. Journal of Cutaneous Pathology. 2004;**31**(2):205-209

[56] Siems W et al. Anti- fibrosclerotic effects of shock wave therapy in lipedema and cellulite. BioFactors. 2005;**24**(1-4):275-282

[57] Sun K et al. Fibrosis and adipose tissue dysfunction. Cell Metabolism. 2013;**18**(4):470-477

[58] Gimble MJ, Katz JA, Bunnell AB. Adipose-derived stem cells for regenerative medicine. Circulation Research. 2007;**100**(9):1249-1260

[59] Gimble JM et al. Concise review: Adipose-derived stromal vascular fraction cells and stem cells: Let's not get lost in translation. 2011: p. 749-754

[60] Uccelli A, Moretta L, Pistoia V. Mesenchymal stem cells in health and disease. Nature Reviews Immunology. 2008;**8**:726

[61] Frese L, Dijkman PE, Hoerstrup SP. Adipose tissue-derived stem cells in regenerative medicine. Transfusion Medicine and Hemotherapy. 2016;**43**(4):268-274

[62] Konno M et al. Adipose-derived mesenchymal stem cells and. Regenerative Medicine. 2013;**55**:309-318

[63] Ong WK, Sugii S. Adipose-derived stem cells: Fatty potentials for therapy. The International Journal of Biochemistry & Cell Biology. 2013;**45**(6):1083

[64] Schneider S. Adipose-derived mesenchymal stem cells from liposuction and resected fat are feasible sources for regenerative medicine. European Journal of Medical Research. 2017;**22**(1):17

[65] Amorin B et al. Mesenchymal stem cell therapy and acute graft-versus-host disease: A review. Human Cell. 2014;**27**:137-150

[66] Li P, Guo X. A review: Therapeutic potential of adipose-derived stem cells in cutaneous wound healing and regeneration. Stem Cell Research & Therapy. 2018;**9**(1)

[67] White IA et al. Mesenchymal stem cells in cardiology. Methods in Molecular Biology (Clifton, N.J.). 2016;**1416**:55

[68] De Francesco F et al. The role of adipose stem cells in inflammatory bowel disease: From biology to novel therapeutic strategies. Cancer Biology & Therapy; 2016. pp. 889-898

[69] Takahashi H et al. Regenerative and transplantation medicine: Cellular therapy using adipose tissue-derived mesenchymal stromal cells for type 1 diabetes mellitus. Journal of Clinical Medicine. 2019;**8**(2):249

[70] Crigna A et al. Stem/stromal cells for treatment of kidney injuries with focus on preclinical models. Frontiers in Medicine. 2018;**5**:179

[71] Paduano F et al. Adipose tissue as a strategic source of mesenchymal stem cells in bone regeneration: A topical review on the most promising craniomaxillofacial applications. International Journal of Molecular Sciences. 2017;**18**(10):2140

[72] Ciuffi S, Zonefrati R, Brandi ML. Adipose stem cells for bone tissue repair. Clinical Cases in Mineral and Bone Metabolism: The Official Journal of the Italian Society of Osteoporosis, Mineral Metabolism, and Skeletal Diseases. 2017;**14**(2):217

[73] Kwak K-A et al. Current perspectives regarding stem cell-based therapy for liver cirrhosis. Canadian Journal of Gastroenterology & Hepatology. 2018;**2018**. Available from: https://doi.org/10.1155/2018/4197857

[74] Bowles AC et al. Adipose stromal vascular fraction attenuates T1 cell-mediated pathology in a model

of multiple sclerosis. Journal of Neuroinflammation. 2018;**15**(1):77

[75] Bourin P et al. Stromal cells from the adipose tissue-derived stromal vascular fraction and culture expanded adipose tissue-derived stromal/stem cells: A joint statement of the International Federation for Adipose Therapeutics and Science (IFATS) and the International Society for Cellular Therapy (ISCT). Cytotherapy. 2013;**15**(6):641

[76] Bunnell BA et al. Adipose-derived stem cells: Isolation, expansion and differentiation. Methods. 2008;**45**(2):115-120

[77] Gnecchi M et al. Paracrine mechanisms of mesenchymal stem cells in tissue repair. Methods in Molecular Biology (Clifton, N.J.). 2016;**1416**:123

[78] Rehman JJ et al. Secretion of angiogenic and antiapoptotic factors by human adipose stromal cells. Circulation: Journal of the American Heart Association. 2004;**109**(10):1292-1298

Chapter 7

Mediators of Impaired Adipogenesis in Obesity-Associated Insulin Resistance and T2DM

Haya Al-Sulaiti, Alexander S. Dömling and Mohamed A. Elrayess

Abstract

Obesity has become a global health issue due to its high prevalence and associated comorbidities including insulin resistance (IR) and type 2 diabetes mellitus (T2DM). Obesity is associated with the expansion of adipose tissues through hypertrophy of mature adipocytes and differentiation of local preadipocytes in a process known as adipogenesis to store excess triacylglycerols (TAGs). Impairment of adipogenesis leads to ectopic fat deposition in skeletal muscles, liver, and kidneys, triggering IR in these tissues and increased risk of T2DM. Many factors contribute to impaired adipogenesis including obesity-associated mild chronic inflammation, oxidative stress, and fatty acid signaling. This review summarizes recent literature covering mediators of impaired adipogenesis and underlying molecular pathways.

Keywords: adipogenesis, mediators, inflammation, oxidative stress, fatty acids

1. Obesity-associated metabolic disease

Rapidly changing lifestyle, accompanied by consumption of excess energy in the form of a calorie-rich high-fat diet, lower voluntary activity, and increased exposure to environmental pollutants, have led to an exponential rise in noncommunicable metabolic diseases [1]. A key component of chronic metabolic diseases is obesity that has become a global health problem associated with a range of comorbidities including insulin resistance and type 2 T2DM [2], coronary artery disease (CAD) [3], nonalcoholic fatty liver [4], cancers [5], and elevated risk of premature death [6, 7].

Adipose tissue is an endocrine organ that responds to obesity by secreting elevated quantities of free fatty acids, adipokines, and proinflammatory cytokines, triggering IR and risk of T2DM [8]. Obesity is also characterized by increased adiposity mediated by enlarged size of mature adipocytes (hypertrophy) and elevated number of newly recruited adipocytes (hyperplasia) [9–12]. Adipose tissue dysfunction is characterized by adipocyte hypertrophy, mild chronic inflammation, and oxidative stress, causing reduced ability to generate new adipocytes from the undifferentiated precursors (preadipocytes). The impaired adipogenesis increases risk of IR and T2DM by triggering ectopic fat deposition in nonadipose tissues

IntechOpen

and proinflammatory environment characterized by impaired secretion of various adipose-derived adipokines [13].

Obesity also represents an imbalance between the primary site of storing energy (the white fat) and the site that is specialized in energy expenditure (the brown fat) [14]. White adipocytes store fat in the form of triacylglycerols as a single fat lipid droplet that gets readily hydrolyzed by lipases when energy is needed. The resulting fatty acids are mobilized to other tissues to undergo fatty acid oxidation as a source of energy [15]. The imbalance between lipolysis and lipogenesis plays a crucial role in progression of metabolic disease including T2DM and nonalcoholic fatty liver disease [16]. The brown fat, on the other hand, uses the energy derived from fatty acid oxidation for heat generation [17].

Adipocyte hypertrophy is associated with increased uptake of excess TAGs, which triggers fat accumulation within the larger subcutaneous adipose tissue (SAT) [18–20]. SAT therefore plays a buffering role as it prohibits progression of obesity-associated pathologies [21]. However, the buffering capacity becomes limited as impairment of SAT expansion causes IR [22–24] as the excess fat are deposited in the visceral adipose tissue (VAT) as well as ectopically in the skeletal muscle, liver, kidney, and heart tissues [25]. This is augmented by the infiltration of macrophages and activation of the innate immune cells [26], which triggers hyperinsulinemia that inhibits lipolysis and activates lipoprotein lipase (LPL). This causes further hyperinsulinemia, hypertriglyceridemia, increased IR in these tissues [27], and risk of T2DM [28].

Although obesity is generally associated with these comorbidities, some obese individuals seem to be protected as they maintain insulin sensitivity (IS) and show lower hypertension and proatherogenic and inflammatory profiles than their equally obese pathogenic counterparts [29–32]. Investigating the underlying causes for this protective phenotype could potentially help obesity-associated pathogenicity. Although still unknown, various potential mechanisms were proposed to contribute to metabolically healthy obese (MHO) phenotype. These include lower visceral and ectopic fat deposition than subcutaneous fat accumulation due to efficient SAT adipogenesis, reduced inflammatory component in the adipose tissue, healthy levels of secreted adipokines, and more active lifestyle [33]. A genetic component was also suggested to interact with various environmental factors, although not yet determined [34]. Interestingly, lean diabetics also exhibit larger adipocytes than healthy individuals, perhaps due to impaired differentiation of preadipocytes but not a result of different frequencies of stromal vascular cells, lipolysis, or levels of inflammatory mediators [35]. Current therapeutic strategies focus on treating obesity-associated diseases instead of preventing the underlying mechanisms. Therefore, understanding the molecular mediators underlying the protective phenotype in MHO individuals could provide critical information to help individuals suffering from pathological obesity (PO). In this review, we aimed to understand the role of adipogenesis in obesity-associated IR and T2DM by screening 2317 articles investigating adipogenesis and mediators of impaired adipogenesis in PubMed with the aid of Rayyne, a systematic review web application [36].

2. The role of adipogenesis in obesity-associated IR and T2DM

The adipose tissue is a dynamic part of the endocrine system that plays a crucial role in maintaining energy balance and nutritional homeostasis [37]. Mature adipocytes constitute the most abundant distinctive cell type in the adipose tissue, occupying 90% of its volume [38]. Other components include leukocytes, macrophages, fibroblasts, endothelial cells, and preadipocytes, which constitute the stromal vascular cells (4–6 million cells per gram of adipose tissue, half of which are immune cells) [39].

Obesity-induced adipocyte hypertrophy is associated with impaired recruitment and differentiation of preadipocytes. Despite their abundance, preadipocytes fail to undergo terminal differentiation into mature adipocytes via the activation of the canonical Wnt signaling [40]. Preadipocytes are produced by mesenchymal stem cells (MSCs) under the influence of different signaling molecules. The mature adipocytes secrete BMP4 that triggers preadipocyte differentiation by inducing the separation of Wnt1 inducible-signaling pathway protein 2 (WISP2) and zinc finger protein 423 (ZNF423), allowing ZNF423 to translocate into the nucleus and activate peroxisome proliferator-activated receptors (PPARγ) and downstream cascade including CCAAT/enhancer-binding proteins β (C/EBPβ), δ, and α [41, 42] (**Figure 1**).

BMP4 also plays an anti-inflammatory role by reducing tumor necrosis factor-α (TNF-α)-mediated proinflammatory cytokine induction in human adipocytes. Therefore, BMP4 plays a protective role against IR and T2DM [43]. Subsequently, PPARγ and C/EBPα activate preadipocyte differentiation and the expression of mature makers such as adiponectin, fatty acid-binding protein 4 (FABP4), glucose transporter type 4 (GLUT4), and LPL. The activation of PPARγ, therefore,

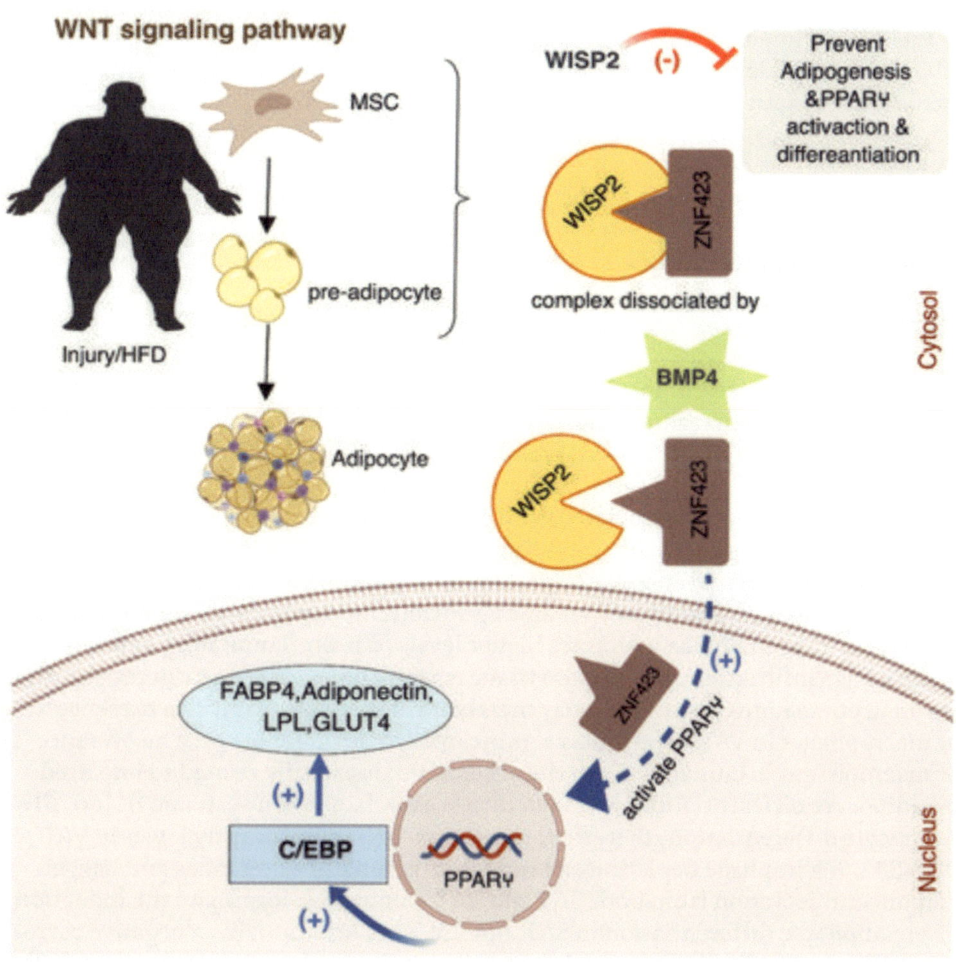

Figure 1.
Schematic representation of the role of Wnt signaling in adipogenesis.

maintains IS and exhibits an anti-inflammatory function, whereas IR causes impaired adipogenesis and increased risk of T2DM [44, 45].

Insulin and downstream Akt signaling also play important roles as modulators of adipose tissue growth and adipogenesis as insulin activates glucose and free fatty acid uptake, inhibits lipolysis, and de novo fatty acid synthesis in adipocytes, and induces adipogenesis [46]. The transcription factor nuclear factor kappa-light-chain-enhancer of activated B cells (NF-κB) has been shown to induce energy expenditure and reduce adipose tissue growth, leading to prevention of dietary obesity and lowering adipogenesis, inflammation, and IR [47]. The inhibition of inhibitor of nuclear factor kappa-B kinase subunit β (IKKβ) in mice lowers high-fat diet-induced adipogenesis and inflammation and protects from diet-induced obesity and IR [48]. MicroRNAs (miRNAs) have been also shown to play an important role in adipogenesis, IR, and inflammation as previously reviewed [49]. Tonicity-responsive enhancer-binding protein (TonEBP), a key transcription factor involved in cellular adaptation to hypertonic stress, has been suggested to influence macrophage activity, adipogenesis, and IS by inhibiting the epigenetic transition of PPARγ2 [50]. Protectin DX (PDX), a ω-3 fatty acid-derived proresolution mediator, was reported to reduce inflammation and IR via an AMPK-dependent pathway and suppress adipogenesis and lipid accumulation during 3T3-L1 differentiation [51].

We have recently shown that higher adipogenic capacity of preadipocytes isolated from SAT and VAT from MHO individuals than PO counterparts may be one of the underlying mechanisms for MHO protection due to a greater ability to store TAGs in the SAT depot. This process was shown to be influenced by inflammatory mediators, oxidative stress, and fatty acid signaling [45, 52–55].

3. Mediators of impaired adipogenesis in IR and T2DM

3.1 Inflammatory mediators

3.1.1 Impaired adipogenesis in response to proinflammatory signals

Obesity-associated comorbidities are mediated by chronic mild inflammation (**Figure 2**). Lipid-laden adipocytes produce increased levels of cytokines such as Interleukin 6 (IL-6), IL-β, TNF-α, monocyte chemoattractant protein-1 (MCP-1), and IL-8 [10, 56, 57] which can inhibit preadipocyte differentiation [21, 45]. The impaired adipogenesis is associated with stress of the endoplasmic reticulum (ER) and elevated expression of unfolded protein response (UPR), both can exacerbate the proinflammatory phenotype of preadipocytes and adipocytes [58]. The effect of proinflammatory phenotype varies among various fat depots. VAT is a more inflammatory tissue than SAT as it secretes higher levels of proinflammatory cytokines. Macrophage infiltration into adipose tissue is regulated through serum resistin and leptin in obese individuals with early metabolic dysfunction [59]. The presence of macrophages in VAT contributes significantly to this phonotype. The presence of macrophages in human SAT, on the other hand, is causally related to impaired preadipocyte differentiation, which in turn is associated with systemic IR [60, 61]. Adipocyte differentiation, therefore, was shown to be significantly lower in VAT than SAT. Macrophage depletion can reduce inflammatory cytokines and trigger adiponectin secretion from both SAT and VAT adipocytes, leading to the induction of preadipocyte differentiation in SAT, but not VAT. Additionally, a negative correlation between SAT adipogenesis, but not VAT, and systemic IR was observed [62]. Chronic systemic inflammation is also associated with elevated lipolysis in white adipose tissue and lipogenesis in nonadipose tissues, causing ectopic fat deposition

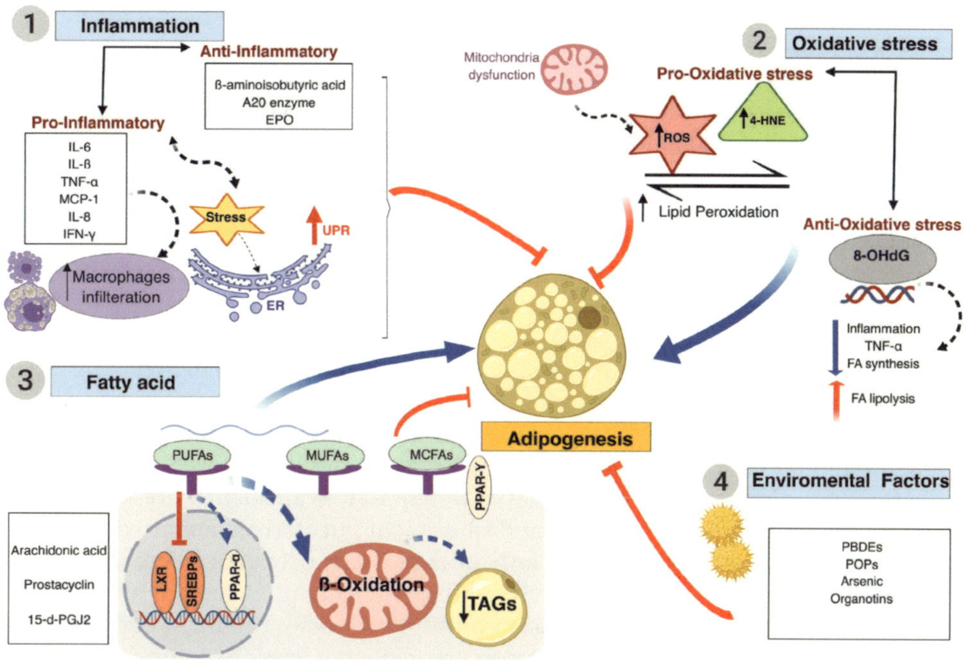

Figure 2.
Mediators of impaired adipogenesis in IR and T2DM. Most proinflammatory cytokines as well as some anti-inflammatory mediators can impair adipogenesis (1). Similarly, various mediators of oxidative stress can impact adipogenesis both positively and negatively depending on their structure (2). Fatty acid signaling plays a key role in adipogenesis but at various degrees depending on the composition of the fatty acids (3). Finally, various environmental factors can impact adipogenesis mostly negatively (4).

in nonadipose tissues and imbalance in free fatty acid homeostasis and increased risk of IR [63].

Among the proinflammatory cytokines, IL-6 is produced by adipocytes, activated leukocytes, and endothelial cells [64] in obesity [65–68]. IL-6 shows a synergistic effect with other mediators of metabolic disease, collectively contributing to the progression of other obesity-associated comorbidities such as CAD and T2DM [64, 69]. IL-6 impairs the LPL function leading to increased levels of circulating fat [69, 70]. Moreover, obesity-associated increase in IL-6 is linked to reduced insulin-triggered glucose uptake [60, 61]. Previous reports have indicated that insulin treatment improves the glucose transport activity of adipocytes in T2DM [21] and lowers IL-6 and TNF-α levels [53]. Although the precise mechanisms of IL-6-associated IR is not well characterized, human adipocytes from IR individuals were shown to exhibit significantly higher IL-6 expression levels [45]. IL-6 impairs insulin action by inhibiting expression of insulin receptor, insulin receptor substrate-1 (IRS-1), and GLUT4 in human preadipocytes as well as 3T3-L1 adipocytes [45, 71]. Furthermore, IL-6 was shown to reduce IS through decrease in adiponectin expression and secretion [72] and via impairment of insulin signaling in hepatocytes [73].

Various other cytokines have been shown to impact adipogenesis [74]. The proinflammatory cytokines IL-1 β, TNF-α, and MCP1 can also influence the hyperplastic expansion of adipose tissue and impair adipogenesis [59]. IL-1β triggers a proinflammatory response in human adipose tissues, particularly in VAT depot. IL-1β also inhibits insulin signal transduction, leading to impaired IS in adipose tissue [75]. IL-1β and cyclooxygenase-2 (COX-2) play a detrimental role in adipose tissue dysfunction in obesity [76]. With obesity, levels of MCP-1 and TNF-α increase in VAT before macrophage infiltration, suggesting a highly proinflammatory phenotype of the visceral depot prior to infiltration of immune cells and macrophage phenotype switch [77]. Unlike IL-6, IL-1 β, and TNF-α, MCP-1 and MCP-1-induced protein (MCPIP) were shown to induce adipogenesis. Treatment of reactive oxygen species (ROS) inhibitor, apocynin, reduced the MCPIP-triggered adipogenesis [78]. Other cytokines involved in adipogenesis include interferon-γ (IFN-γ), a central mediator of macrophage function. Compared to obese wild-type control animals, obese IFN-γ knockouts exhibit better IS, smaller adipocyte size, and lower cytokine expression [79].

3.1.2 Impaired adipogenesis in response to anti-inflammatory signals

Contrary to the notion that inflammation plays a negative role in metabolism, some studies suggest that proinflammatory signals in the adipocytes are actually needed for functional adipose tissue homeostasis (**Figure 2**). Indeed, adipose tissue inflammation was shown in various animal models of adipose tissue-specific reduction of proinflammatory potential to be required as an adaptive response, allowing proper storage of excess fat and filtering of gut-derived endotoxins [80]. Additionally, various molecules with anti-inflammatory properties were shown to influence adipogenesis and risk of IR. Myokines, for example, secreted by skeletal muscle cells during exercise such as β-aminoisobutyric acid, can impair adipogenesis via activating AMPK signaling pathway and reducing levels of proinflammatory cytokines such as TNF-α [81]. Another example is the ubiquitin-editing enzyme A20 that impairs IL-6 secretion from adipocytes, leading to modulation of differentiation of MSCs [82]. The overexpression of A20 was also shown to reduce lipogenesis and adipogenesis via lowering levels of sterol regulatory element binding protein-1c (SREBP-1c) and aP2, causing lower fat accumulation in differentiated 3T3-L1 cells [83]. A third example is the nonerythropoietic EPO-derived peptide that plays an anti-inflammatory and anti-adipogenic roles in high-fat die mice with IR [84]. On the other hand, other anti-inflammatory molecules could rescue impaired adipogenesis. Glucose-dependent insulinotropic polypeptide (GIP), for example, is a potent activator of adipogenesis through modulation of inflammation in adipose tissue [85]. Additionally, the expression of neuronatin (Nnat), a proteolipid involved in neuronal development, in response to inflammation and dietary excess, has been suggested to play an important role in adipogenesis through lowering oxidative stress and inflammation [86].

3.2 Oxidative stress

Obesity leads to the accumulation of ROS, the hallmark of oxidative stress, in the adipose tissue causing impaired adipogenesis and increased risk of IR and T2DM. The balance between ROS generation and activation of endogenous antioxidants is crucial for cells undergoing adipogenesis [87] (**Figure 2**). The oxidative damage and changes in the expression of antioxidant enzymes with age are similar between SAT and VAT. However, preadipocytes from SAT are significantly more resistant than VAT-derived cells to cell death caused by oxidative stress [88]. Interestingly, within SAT and VAT depots, preadipocytes from insulin-sensitive obese subjects were more prone to oxidative damage than preadipocytes from equally obese insulin-resistant individuals [52, 53]. The depletion of ROS from adipose tissue in mice models of oxidative stress was associated with increased adipose tissue mass, lower ectopic fat deposition, and enhanced IS. Similarly, ROS accumulation limited the expansion of adipose tissue, leading to elevated ectopic fat accumulation and increased risk of IR [89]. Elevated ROS within the adipose tissue triggers lipid peroxidation [45] and accumulation of reactive aldehydes including the bioactive lipid peroxidation product 4-hydroxynonenal (4-HNE) [90]. Elevated 4-HNE causes damage of cell structure and function through the formation of the stable adducts 4-hydroxyalkenals with proteins, phospholipids, and DNA [91, 92]. Increased 4-HNE levels have been associated with impaired adipogenesis and IR [53, 93–96]. Another marker of oxidative damage is 8-hydroxy-2-deoxyguanosine (8-OHdG) which was recently shown to exert anti-inflammatory effects, by reducing TNF-α-induced IR in vitro. It was also shown to reduce adipose tissue mass in vivo through activation of adipose triglyceride lipase and lowering the expression of fatty acid synthase [97]. Levels of cholesterol oxidation-derived oxysterols increase in adipose tissues of T2DM patients and act as inhibitors of adipogenesis through activation of Wnt pathway [98]. Heme oxygenase (HO), a major cytoprotective enzyme, functions upstream of Wnt signaling and lowers lipogenesis and adipogenesis, decreasing lipid accumulation and levels of proinflammatory cytokines [99].

Conversely, ROS was also shown to enhance adipogenesis by lowering sirtuin 1 (Sirt1) expression [100, 101]. Heme-induced oxidative stress was shown to inhibit Sirt1, leading to increased adipogenesis [102]. The expression of deleted in bladder cancer protein 1 (DBC1), another inhibitor of the Sirt1, is reduced with obesity, leading to lower adipogenesis and VAT dysfunction [103]. Sirt3 plays a crucial role in mitochondrial function. Silencing of Sirt3 can cause adipocyte dysfunction which impairs adipogenesis and causes IR [104]. Nonselenocysteine-containing phospholipid hydroperoxide glutathione peroxidase (NPGPx) is a sensor of oxidative stress. Lack of NPGPx causes elevation in ROS and promotion of adipogenesis through ROS-dependent dimerization of protein kinase A regulatory subunits and activation of C/EBPβ [105]. Additional evidence suggesting ROS involvement in promotion of adipogenesis comes from antioxidant supplementation experiments where lower levels of ROS resulting from antioxidants contribute to adipose tissue dysfunction and IR [106]. Indeed, antioxidant supplementation exhibited a negative impact when used before induction of oxidative stress as a result of lowering physiological ROS levels because ROS plays a role as second messengers in adipogenesis, lipid metabolism, and insulin signaling [107]. For example, the supplementation with N-acetylcysteine, a known antioxidant and precursor of glutathione, was shown to reduce fat deposition during adipogenic differentiation of mouse fibroblasts [108]. Activation of beta-3 adrenergic receptor (β3-AR) enhances ROS accumulation in cultured adipocytes. Antioxidants enhance β3-AR-triggered mitochondrial ROS production, suggesting that chronic supplementation of antioxidants could indeed generate an elevation in oxidative stress associated with mitochondrial dysfunction in adipocyte [109]. On the other hand, glutathione depletion was shown to inhibit adipogenesis as the result of lowering cell proliferation during the initial mitotic clonal expansion of the adipocyte differentiation process [110].

3.3 Fatty acid signaling

The main role of adipocytes is TAG storage. Although TAGs do not function as signaling molecules per se, the lipid intermediates generated during lipogenesis and lipolysis influence intracellular insulin signaling and participate in progression of IR. These include free fatty acids, diacylglycerols (DAGs), and ceramides [111].

Lipolysis-driven efflux of fatty acids triggers TAG synthesis and causes stress of the ER and activation of June kinase pathway in the adipose tissues [112, 113]. This leads to an elevation in the levels of both DAGs and ceramides and progression of IR in adipocytes [114]. Ceramides were shown to influence lipid-mediated IR in muscles. Delta 4-desaturase, sphingolipid 1 (DEGS1) is a desaturase that mediates ceramide biosynthetic pathway. Ablation of DEGS1 in preadipocytes prevented adipogenesis and decreased lipid accumulation [115]. There are essential enzymes responsible for TAG hydrolysis including hormone-sensitive lipase (HSL), adipose triglyceride lipase (ATGL), and monoglyceride lipase (MGL) [116]. ATGL regulates lipolysis by transcription factor specificity protein 1 (Sp1). Insulin-mediated transcription of Sp1 is critical for this regulation. In mature adipocytes, PPARγ reverses transcriptional repression by Sp1 at the ATGL promoter, leading to stimulation of ATGL mRNA expression. During obesity and IR, the transcription of ATGL becomes downregulated. The extent of the downregulation depends on interactions between Sp1 and PPARγ [117].

A number of factors influence the function of fatty acids in regulating adipogenesis. The number of carbons and the position and number of double bounds are crucial determinants of properties of the fatty acids. Changes in fatty acids including elongation, desaturation, β-oxidation, peroxidation, and incorporation into phospo- and complex lipids can play an essential role in their metabolic function. Fatty acids and their metabolites can control protein expression involved in lipid and energy metabolism by influencing gene transcription, mRNA processing, and posttranslational modifications [118–121]. Most fatty acids activate all three members of the PPAR family [122–125]. Polyunsaturated fatty acids (PUFAs), except for erucic acid, are more potent stimulators of PPARγ than monounsaturated fatty acids (MUFAs) and saturated fatty acids [122–126] (**Figure 2**). The optimal binding affinity is reached with 16–20 carbon-containing compounds. DHA too was shown to stimulate PPARs [124]. Various studies have reported the beneficial effects of PUFAs on lipid-related human disorders [127–131], which largely depend on the structure of the fatty acids and their metabolic properties. PUFAs can inhibit lipogenic gene transcription by downregulating the expression SREBPs [132–135] and act as antagonists of liver X receptors (LXR) [136, 137] and as agonists for PPARs [122–124, 138, 139]. PUFAs, but not saturated or MUFAs, inhibit lipogenic genes by downregulating SREBP-1c. PPAR alpha plays an important role in metabolic adaptation to fasting by enhancing mitochondrial and peroxisomal fatty acid oxidation and ketogenesis [140]. Dietary PUFAs were also shown to stimulate expression of PPARα target genes, induce β-oxidation, and lower plasma TAGs [141–149]. Fatty acids can also play a role as modulators of kinase signaling pathways [150–155].

Arachidonic acid (AA), a polyunsaturated omega-6 fatty acid, is the major PUFA that has been implicated in the regulation of adipogenesis. Short exposure of 3T3-L1 mouse preadipocytes to AA triggers adipocyte differentiation, associated with increase in (FABP4/aP2). Calcium, protein kinase C, and ERK play critical role in this pathway through which AA induces the expression of adipocyte protein 2 (aP2) [156]. AA binds to PPAR-γ2 to stimulate GLUT4 expression in HepG2 cell line, exhibiting an alternative insulin-independent activation of GLUT4 [157]. AA cascade is then controlled by cyclooxygenases enzymes, lipoxygenases, and P450 epoxygenases. When AA is generated from plasma membrane via phospholipases and then metabolized by prostaglandin G/H synthase, different prostaglandins are produced, causing opposing effects on adipocyte differentiation. The proadipogenic effect of AA is mediated by prostaglandin product (prostacyclin) and is thus cyclooxygenase dependent [158–160]. Among prostaglandin classes, 15-deoxy-Δ12,14-prostaglandin J2 (15-d-PGJ2) was shown to be proadipogenic [161, 162]. On the other hand, prostaglandin F2α (PGF2α) was shown to exert anti-adipogenic effects in primary preadipocytes [163–165], 1246 cells [164], and 3T3-L1 cells [166–168]. The anti-adipogenic effect of PGF2α is mediated through prostaglandin F receptor-mediated elevation in intracellular calcium and DNA synthesis [168] and activation of MAPK, causing reduction in PPARγ phosphorylation [169]. The role of prostaglandin E2 (PGE2), the third main prostaglandin, in adipogenesis is controversial as PGE2 exhibits antilipolytic effect in mature adipocytes but shows no effect on preadipocytes [170]. However, it was recently demonstrated that PGE2 inhibited adipogenesis of 3T3-L1 cells [171, 172]. Epoxyeicosatrienoic acids (EETs), AA metabolites, and AA-derived cytochrome P450 (CYP) epoxygenase metabolites exert anti-inflammatory effects in the vasculature. The expression of CYP2J, a member of P450 subfamily with a role in the bioactivation of AA in extrahepatic tissues, inhibits NF-κB and MAPK signaling pathways and activates of PPARγ, thus reducing IR and diabetic phenotype [173]. n-3 PUFAs, on the other hand, reduce adipose growth and play a role in adipogenesis in various rodent studies [174–183].

Medium-chain fatty acids (MCFAs) (C8–C10) bind the PPARγ ligand binding domain in vitro, causing full inhibition of phosphorylation of PPARγ by cyclin-dependent kinase 5 (cdk5) and reversal of IR in adipose tissue. MCFAs that bind PPARγ also inhibit thiazolidinedione-dependent adipogenesis in vitro [184]. On the other hand, MUFAs were shown to induce adipogenesis and enhance TAG accumulation in 3T3-L1 mouse preadipocytes. Levels of TAGs were greater in cells treated with c-22:1 than c18:1 and c-20:1. Among the c-22:1 fatty acids, c9–22:1 treatment showed higher fat accumulation, associated with increased expression of adipogenic and lipogenic transcription factors, such as PPARγ and C/EBPα and SREBP-1. However, c-20:1 FAs exhibited less effect than c-18:1 and c-22:1 [185]. Alpha-lipoic acid (ALA) activates insulin signaling pathway and exerts insulin-like properties in adipose and muscle cells. However, 3T3-L1 preadipocytes treated with LA exhibit lower insulin-induced differentiation by modulating activity and/or expression of various anti-adipogenic transcription factors mainly through activating the MAPK pathways that negatively regulate PPARγ and C/EBPα [141]. 10-oxo-12(Z)-octadecenoic acid, a linoleic acid metabolite, triggered adipocyte differentiation through PPARγ activation and elevated adiponectin secretion and insulin-triggered glucose uptake [142]. Dietary n-3 fatty acids showed more effective activation of PPARα in the liver of rodents [143–145] than n-6 fatty acids [146]. **Figure 3** summarizes the

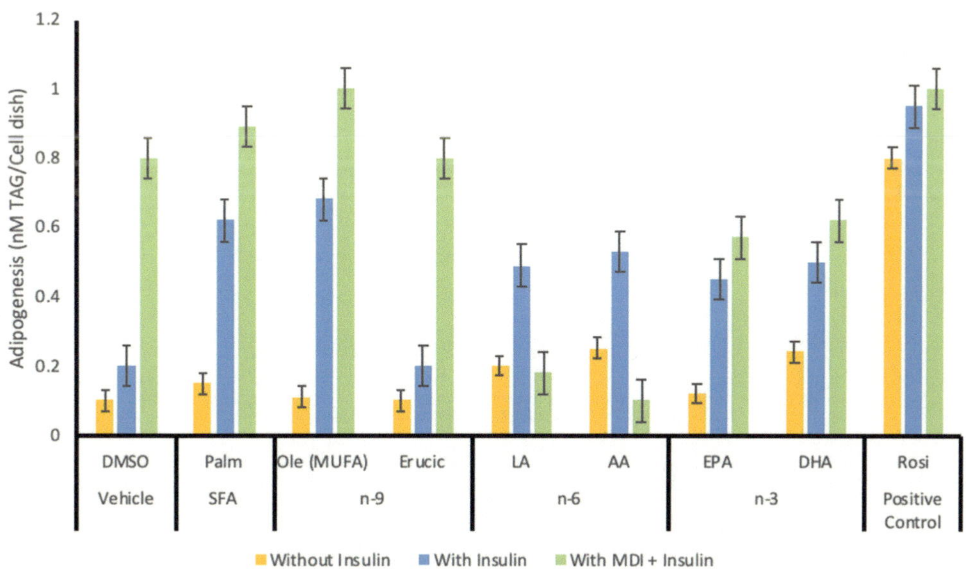

Figure 3.
Adipogenic capacity of various fatty acids in 3T3L-1 cells in the absence or presence of 1 μg/ml insulin in differentiation medium (MDI) containing 0.5 mM isobutyl-1-methylxanthine and 1 μM dexamethasone in DMEM and 10% FBS. 100 μM palmitic acid (palm), oleic acid (ole), erucic acid, linoleic acid (LA), arachidonic acid (AA), eicosapentaenoic acid (EPA), docosahexaenoic acid (DHA), or 1 μM rosiglitazone (rosi) dissolved in DMSO were added when differentiation was induced at day 0 and were present throughout the differentiation period (adapted from Madsen et al.) [147].

effect of various fatty acid species on the proadipogenic capacity of 3T3L-1 cells in the presence or absence of insulin (Madsen et al.) [147].

Lipidomics studies were performed to investigate differences between SAT and VAT depots. These studies have shown evidence of depot-specific enrichment of certain species of TAGs, glycerophospholipids, and sphingolipids and specific correlations between certain lipid species and body mass index, inflammation, and IS [148, 149]. We have recently shown in human SAT and omental (OM) adipose tissue biopsies from 64 obese individuals a number of TAGs that changed with increased risk IR and T2DM including C46:4, C48:5, C48:4, C38:1, C50:3, C40:2, C56:3, C56:4, C56:7, and C58:7. Enrichment analysis showed C12:0 fatty acid to be associated with TAGs that are least abundant in T2DM. Our data also indicated that C18:3 was present in both depleted and enriched TAGs in T2DM [55]. Secretion of interleukin IL-6 was found to be significantly lower after treatment with C18:2, C22:6, and C16:0 through blocking NF-κB and activating PPARγ [186]. Our data also showed positive correlations between C56:4 and C57:4, both containing C18:2 and C16:0, with SC adipogenic capacity. OM adipogenic capacity was associated with C49:1, C38:0, and C56:2, containing C16:0, C18:1, and C14:0 [55]. **Table 1** summarizes a list of

Metabolic trait	R^2	Importance	TAG	MW	Fatty acid composition	Fatty acid identities
SC adipogenic	0.9	0.16	C58:10	926.8	C18:2, C18:2, C22:6	Linoleic acid, linoleic acid, docosahexaenoic acid
		0.16	C56:4	910.8	C18:1, C18:2, C20:1	Oleic acid, linoleic acid, gadoleic acid
		0.14	C57:4	924.7	C22:0, C19:4, C16:0	Behenic acid, C19:4, palmitic acid
		0.09	C40:1	692.7	C18:1, C16:0, C6:0	Oleic acid, palmitic acid, caproic acid
		0.08	C60:1	970.8	C24:0, C24:0, C18:1	Lignoceric acid, oleic acid
		0.22	C38:1	664.7	C18:1, C16:0, C4:0	Oleic acid, palmitic acid, butyric acid
OM adipogenic	1	0.18	C48:1	804.8	C18:0, C16:1, C14:0	Stearic acid, palmitoleic acid, myristic acid
		0.14	C49:1	818.7	C18:1, C17:0, C14:0	Oleic acid, heptadecanoic acid, myristic acid
		0.11	C56:1	916.8	C18:0, C18:0, C20:1	Stearic acid, stearic acid, gadoleic
		0.09	C54:0	890.8	C18:0, C18:0, C18:0	Stearic acid, stearic acid
		0.06	C38:0	666.7	C10:0, C14:0, C14:0	Capric acid, myristic acid
		0.05	C56:2	914.8	C18:1, C18:1, C20:0	Oleic acid, oleic acid, arachidic acid
		0.04	C51:1	846.7	C18:1, C15:0, C18:0	Oleic acid, pentadecanoic acid, stearic acid

Table 1.
List of TAGs associated with IR, SC, and OM adipogenic capacity.

TAGs associated with SAT and OM adipogenic capacity. These fatty acids were reported to stimulate adipogenesis in rodents [187–191] and potentially in human preadipocytes.

4. Environmental factors

Various types of environmental factors were shown to influence adipogenesis. These include environmental pollutants. Among the environmental pollutants, polybrominated diphenyl ethers (PBDEs) represent a widely used type of flame retardants in commercial products and a main source of environmental contaminants. PBDEs accumulate in adipose tissue, potentially changing its endocrine function causing elevation in the risk of IR. We have previously shown that specific congeners of PBDEs (28, 47, 99, and 153) were predominant in VAT from obese individuals and that PBDEs 99, 28, and 47 were elevated in obese IR compared to obese IS. Treatment of human VAT-derived preadipocytes from obese IS individuals with PBDE28 inhibited insulin signaling and reduced adipogenesis [54]. In addition to PBDEs, evidence linking accumulation of other persistent organic pollutants (POPs) and risk of IR and T2DM was previously described [54, 192]. Additionally, the association between inorganic arsenic exposure and the risk of T2DM and obesity was previously reported [193]. Arsenic-induced T2DM is suggested to be mediated by inflammation, oxidative stress, and apoptosis, playing a significant role in the pathogenesis of obesity. Arsenic inhibits adipogenesis and enhances lipolysis, leading to obesity. Other reports have suggested that arsenic may induce lipodystrophy [193]. Another evidence suggests that uremic toxin-treated 3T3-L1 cells and MSC-derived adipocytes exhibit impaired adipogenesis and apoptosis through activation of the Na/K-ATPase/ROS amplification cycle [194]. Other types of environmental pollutants include organotins, widely used antifouling biocides for ships and fishing nets, play a role as endocrine disruptors as they bind to PPARγ/RXRα, induce adipogenesis, and repress inflammatory genes in different mammalian cells [195].

5. Conclusion

The pathology of obesity-associated IR and T2DM involves ectopic fat deposition in response to elevated energy intake and poor fat storage. The latter is due to impaired adipogenesis as newly recruited preadipocytes become unable to differentiate into fully functional adipocytes. This review presents several factors that influence adipogenesis in pathological obesity including inflammatory mediators, oxidative stress, fatty acid signaling, and other environmental factors. Most proinflammatory cytokines such as IL-6, IL-1β, TNF-α, IL-8, and IFNγ as well as some anti-inflammatory mediators including β-aminoisobutyric acid, A20 enzyme, and EPO have been shown to impair adipogenesis, leading to adipocyte hypertrophy, ectopic fat accumulation, and increased risk of IR and T2DM. However, basal level of adipose tissue inflammation has been shown to be required for normal adipogenesis and functional adipose tissue homeostasis. Similarly, various mediators of oxidative stress were shown to impact adipogenesis positively such as lipid peroxidation product 4-HNE and negatively such as the marker of oxidative damage 8-OHdG. Targeting lipid peroxidation products was shown to reverse impairment of adipogenesis and sustain IS. However, complete depletion of oxidative stress could also lead to impairment of adipogenesis as basal oxidative stress was shown to be required for normal adipogenesis. Fatty acid signaling also plays a very important role in adipogenesis as various fatty acid species such as PUFAs, MUFAs, and MCFAs were shown to regulate preadipocyte differentiation at various degrees depending on their composition. Finally, various environmental factors were suggested to impact adipogenesis, mainly through triggering inflammation and oxidative stress, leading to impairment of adipogenesis and increased risk of IR.

Competing interests

The authors declare that they have no competing interests.

Authors' contributions

All authors participated in reviewing the literature and preparing and approving the manuscript. MAE is responsible for the integrity of the work as a whole.

Abbreviations

COX-2	cyclooxygenase-2
15-d-PGJ2	15-deoxy-Δ12,14-prostaglandin J2
4-HNE	4-hydroxynonenal
8-OHdG	8-hydroxy-2-deoxyguanosine
AA	arachidonic acid
ATGL	adipose triglyceride lipase
BMP4	bone morphogenetic protein 4
C/EBP	CCAAT/enhancer-binding protein
CAD	Coronary artery disease
cdk5	cyclin-dependent kinase 5
DAGs	diacylglycerols
DBC1	deleted in bladder cancer protein 1
DHA	docosahexaenoic acid
DMEM	dexamethasone
DMSO	dimethyl sulfoxide
EETs	epoxyeicosatrienoic acids
EPA	eicosapentaenoic acid
EPO	nonerythropoietic derived peptide
ER	endoplasmic reticulum
FABP4	fatty acid-binding protein 4
GIP	glucose-dependent insulinotropic polypeptide
HSL	hormone-sensitive lipase
IFN-γ	interferon-γ
IKKβ	inhibitor of nuclear factor kappa-B kinase subunit β
IL-6	interleukin 6
IR	insulin resistance
IS	insulin sensitive
LA	linoleic acid
LPL	lipoprotein lipase
LXR	liver X receptors
MCFAs	medium chain fatty acids
MCP-1	monocyte chemoattractant protein-1
MCPIP	Mcp-1-induced protein

MDI	insulin in differentiation medium
MGL	monoglyceride lipase
MHO	metabolically healthy obese
miRNAs	microRNAs
MUFAs	monounsaturated fatty acids
NF-kappa-B	nuclear factor kappa-light-chain enhancer of activated B cells
Nnat	neurontin
NPGPx	nonselenocysteine-containing phospholipid hydroperoxide glutathione peroxidase
Ole	oleic acid
OM	omental adipose tissue
Palm	palmitic acid
PBDEs	diphenyl ethers
PDX	protectin DX
PGE2	prostaglandin E2
PGF2α	prostaglandin F2α
PO	pathological obesity
POPs	organic pollutants
PPAR	peroxisome proliferator-activated receptors
PUFAs	polyunsaturated fatty acids
ROS	reactive oxygen species
Rosi	rosiglitazone
SAT	subcutaneous adipose tissue
Sirt1	sirtuin 1
Sp1	transcription factor specificity protein 1
SREBP-1c	sterol regulatory element binding protein 1C
T2DM	type 2 diabetes
TAGs	triacylglycerolsTNF-α tumor necrosis factor-α
TonEBP	tonicity-responsive enhancer-binding protein
UPR	unfolded protein response
VAT	visceral adipose tissue
WISP2	inducible-signaling pathway protein 2
ZNF423	zinc finger protein 423
β3-AR	beta-3 adrenergic receptor
MSCs	mesenchymal stem cells
Ap2	adipocyte protein 2
CYP	cytochrome P450
ALA	alpha-lipoic acid

Author details

Haya Al-Sulaiti[1], Alexander S. Dömling[1] and Mohamed A. Elrayess[2*]

1 Department of Drug Design, University of Groningen, Groningen, Netherlands

2 Biomedical Research Center (BRC), Qatar University, Doha, Qatar

*Address all correspondence to: maelrayess@hotmail.com

References

[1] Maire B et al. Nutritional transition and non-communicable diet-related chronic diseases in developing countries. Santé. 2002;**12**(1):45-55

[2] Kodama S et al. Quantitative relationship between body weight gain in adulthood and incident type 2 diabetes: A meta-analysis. Obesity Reviews. 2014;**15**(3):202-214

[3] Bogers RP et al. Association of overweight with increased risk of coronary heart disease partly independent of blood pressure and cholesterol levels: A meta-analysis of 21 cohort studies including more than 300 000 persons. Archives of Internal Medicine. 2007;**167**(16):1720-1728

[4] Tsuneto A et al. Fatty liver incidence and predictive variables. Hypertension Research. 2010;**33**(6):638-643

[5] Eliassen AH et al. Adult weight change and risk of postmenopausal breast cancer. Journal of the American Medical Association. 2006;**296**(2):193-201

[6] McGee DL, Diverse Populations C. Body mass index and mortality: A meta-analysis based on person-level data from twenty-six observational studies. Annals of Epidemiology. 2005;**15**(2):87-97

[7] Adams KF et al. Overweight, obesity, and mortality in a large prospective cohort of persons 50 to 71 years old. The New England Journal of Medicine. 2006;**355**(8):763-778

[8] Makki K, Froguel P, Wolowczuk I. Adipose tissue in obesity-related inflammation and insulin resistance: Cells, cytokines, and chemokines. ISRN Inflammation. 2013;**2013**:139239

[9] Jo J et al. Hypertrophy and/or hyperplasia: Dynamics of adipose tissue growth. PLoS Computational Biology. 2009;**5**(3):e1000324

[10] Bjorntorp P. Effects of age, sex, and clinical conditions on adipose tissue cellularity in man. Metabolism. 1974;**23**(11):1091-1102

[11] Spalding KL et al. Dynamics of fat cell turnover in humans. Nature. 2008;**453**(7196):783-787

[12] Rutkowski JM, Stern JH, Scherer PE. The cell biology of fat expansion. The Journal of Cell Biology. 2015;**208**(5):501-512

[13] Murdolo G et al. Oxidative stress and lipid peroxidation by-products at the crossroad between adipose organ dysregulation and obesity-linked insulin resistance. Biochimie. 2013;**95**(3):585-594

[14] Elattar S, Satyanarayana A. Can brown fat win the battle against white fat? Journal of Cellular Physiology. 2015;**230**(10):2311-2317

[15] Ahmadian M, Wang Y, Sul HS. Lipolysis in adipocytes. The International Journal of Biochemistry and Cell Biology. 2010;**42**(5):555-559

[16] Saponaro C et al. The subtle balance between lipolysis and lipogenesis: A critical point in metabolic homeostasis. Nutrients. 2015;**7**(11):9453-9474

[17] Rosen ED, Spiegelman BM. Adipocytes as regulators of energy balance and glucose homeostasis. Nature. 2006;**444**(7121):847-853

[18] Okuno A et al. Troglitazone increases the number of small adipocytes without the change of white adipose tissue mass in obese Zucker rats. The Journal of Clinical Investigation. 1998;**101**(6):1354-1361

[19] Tontonoz P, Hu E, Spiegelman BM. Stimulation of adipogenesis in

fibroblasts by PPAR gamma 2, a lipid-activated transcription factor. Cell. 1994;**79**(7):1147-1156

[20] Cinti S et al. Adipocyte death defines macrophage localization and function in adipose tissue of obese mice and humans. Journal of Lipid Research. 2005;**46**(11):2347-2355

[21] Radcke S, Dillon JF, Murray AL. A systematic review of the prevalence of mildly abnormal liver function tests and associated health outcomes. European Journal of Gastroenterology and Hepatology. 2015;**27**(1):1-7

[22] Vigouroux C et al. Molecular mechanisms of human lipodystrophies: From adipocyte lipid droplet to oxidative stress and lipotoxicity. The International Journal of Biochemistry and Cell Biology. 2011;**43**(6):862-876

[23] Virtue S, Vidal-Puig A. Adipose tissue expandability, lipotoxicity and the metabolic syndrome—An allostatic perspective. Biochimica et Biophysica Acta. 2010;**1801**(3):338-349

[24] Xue P et al. Adipose deficiency of Nrf2 in Ob/Ob mice results in severe metabolic syndrome. Diabetes. 2013;**62**(3):845-854

[25] Hocking S et al. Adiposity and insulin resistance in humans: The role of the different tissue and cellular lipid depots. Endocrine Reviews. 2013;**34**(4):463-500

[26] Kursawe R et al. A role of the inflammasome in the low storage capacity of the abdominal subcutaneous adipose tissue in obese adolescents. Diabetes. 2016;**65**(3):610-618

[27] Snel M et al. Ectopic fat and insulin resistance: Pathophysiology and effect of diet and lifestyle interventions. International Journal of Endocrinology. 2012;**2012**:983814

[28] Guilherme A et al. Adipocyte dysfunctions linking obesity to insulin resistance and type 2 diabetes. Nature Reviews. Molecular Cell Biology. 2008;**9**(5):367-377

[29] Bogardus C et al. Relationship between degree of obesity and in vivo insulin action in man. The American Journal of Physiology. 1985;**248**(3 Pt 1): E286-E291

[30] Samocha-Bonet D et al. Insulin-sensitive obesity in humans—A 'favorable fat' phenotype? Trends in Endocrinology and Metabolism. 2012;**23**(3):116-124

[31] Karelis AD et al. The metabolically healthy but obese individual presents a favorable inflammation profile. The Journal of Clinical Endocrinology and Metabolism. 2005;**90**(7):4145-4150

[32] Stefan N et al. Identification and characterization of metabolically benign obesity in humans. Archives of Internal Medicine. 2008;**168**(15):1609-1616

[33] Stefan N et al. Metabolically healthy obesity: Epidemiology, mechanisms, and clinical implications. The Lancet Diabetes and Endocrinology. 2013;**1**(2):152-162

[34] Jung CH, Lee WJ, Song KH. Metabolically healthy obesity: A friend or foe? The Korean Journal of Internal Medicine. 2017;**32**(4):611-621

[35] Acosta JR et al. Increased fat cell size: A major phenotype of subcutaneous white adipose tissue in non-obese individuals with type 2 diabetes. Diabetologia. 2016;**59**(3):560-570

[36] Ouzzani M et al. Rayyan-a web and mobile app for systematic reviews. Systematic Reviews. 2016;**5**(1):210

[37] Coelho M, Oliveira T, Fernandes R. Biochemistry of adipose tissue: An

endocrine organ. Archives of Medical Science. 2013;**9**(2):191-200

[38] Yuan Y, Gao J, Ogawa R. Mechanobiology and mechanotherapy of adipose tissue-effect of mechanical force on fat tissue engineering. Plastic and Reconstructive Surgery. Global Open. 2015;**3**(12):e578

[39] Han S et al. Adipose-derived stromal vascular fraction cells: Update on clinical utility and efficacy. Critical Reviews in Eukaryotic Gene Expression. 2015;**25**(2):145-152

[40] Gustafson B et al. Restricted adipogenesis in hypertrophic obesity: The role of WISP2, WNT, and BMP4. Diabetes. 2013;**62**(9):2997-3004

[41] Hammarstedt A et al. WISP2 regulates preadipocyte commitment and PPAR gamma activation by BMP4. Proceedings of the National Academy of Sciences of the United States of America. 2013;**110**(7):2563-2568

[42] Gupta RK et al. Transcriptional control of preadipocyte determination by Zfp423. Nature. 2010;**464**(7288):619-623

[43] Baraban E et al. Anti-inflammatory properties of bone morphogenetic protein 4 in human adipocytes. International Journal of Obesity (2005). 2016;**40**(2):319-327

[44] Gustafson B et al. Insulin resistance and impaired adipogenesis. Trends in Endocrinology and Metabolism. 2015;**26**(4):193-200

[45] Almuraikhy S et al. Interleukin-6 induces impairment in human subcutaneous adipogenesis in obesity-associated insulin resistance. Diabetologia. 2016;**59**(11):2406-2416

[46] Peng X et al. Thioredoxin reductase 1 suppresses adipocyte differentiation and insulin responsiveness. Scientific Reports. 2016;**6**:28080

[47] Tang T et al. Uncoupling of inflammation and insulin resistance by NF-kappaB in transgenic mice through elevated energy expenditure. The Journal of Biological Chemistry. 2010;**285**(7):4637-4644

[48] Helsley RN et al. Targeting IκB kinase β in adipocyte lineage cells for treatment of obesity and metabolic dysfunctions. Stem Cells (Dayton, Ohio). 2016;**34**(7):1883-1895

[49] Hilton C, Neville MJ, Karpe F. MicroRNAs in adipose tissue: Their role in adipogenesis and obesity. International Journal of Obesity (2005). 2013;**37**(3):325-332

[50] Lee JH et al. TonEBP suppresses adipogenesis and insulin sensitivity by blocking epigenetic transition of PPARγ2. Scientific Reports. 2015;**5**:10937

[51] Jung TW et al. Protectin DX attenuates LPS-induced inflammation and insulin resistance in adipocytes via AMPK-mediated suppression of the NF-κB pathway. American Journal of Physiology. Endocrinology and Metabolism. 2018;**315**(4):E543-E551

[52] Elrayess MA et al. 4-hydroxynonenal causes impairment of human subcutaneous adipogenesis and induction of adipocyte insulin resistance. Free Radical Biology and Medicine. 2017;**104**:129-137

[53] Jaganjac M et al. Combined metformin and insulin treatment reverses metabolically impaired omental adipogenesis and accumulation of 4-hydroxynonenal in obese diabetic patients. Redox Biology. 2017;**12**:483-490

[54] Helaleh M et al. Association of polybrominated diphenyl ethers in two fat compartments with increased risk of insulin resistance in obese individuals. Chemosphere. 2018;**209**:268-276

[55] Al-Sulaiti H et al. Triglyceride profiling in adipose tissues from obese insulin sensitive, insulin resistant and type 2 diabetes mellitus individuals. Journal of Translational Medicine. 2018;**16**(1):175

[56] Acosta JR et al. Increased fat cell size: A major phenotype of subcutaneous white adipose tissue in non-obese individuals with type 2 diabetes. Diabetologia. 2016;**59**(3):560-570

[57] Flower L et al. Stimulation of interleukin-6 release by interleukin-1beta from isolated human adipocytes. Cytokine. 2003;**21**(1):32-37

[58] Longo M et al. Pathologic endoplasmic reticulum stress induced by glucotoxic insults inhibits adipocyte differentiation and induces an inflammatory phenotype. Biochimica et Biophysica Acta. 2016;**1863**(6 Pt A): 1146-1156

[59] Kang YE et al. The roles of adipokines, proinflammatory cytokines, and adipose tissue macrophages in obesity-associated insulin resistance in modest obesity and early metabolic dysfunction. PLoS One. 2016;**11**(4):e0154003

[60] Kern PA et al. Adipose tissue tumor necrosis factor and interleukin-6 expression in human obesity and insulin resistance. American Journal of Physiology. Endocrinology and Metabolism. 2001;**280**(5):E745-E751

[61] Fasshauer M et al. Interleukin (IL)-6 mRNA expression is stimulated by insulin, isoproterenol, tumour necrosis factor alpha, growth hormone, and IL-6 in 3T3-L1 adipocytes. Hormone and Metabolic Research. 2003;**35**(3):147-152

[62] Liu LF et al. Adipose tissue macrophages impair preadipocyte differentiation in humans. PLoS One. 2017;**12**(2):e0170728

[63] Mei M et al. Inflammatory stress exacerbates ectopic lipid deposition in C57BL/6J mice. Lipids in Health and Disease. 2011;**10**:110

[64] Pradhan AD et al. C-reactive protein, interleukin 6, and risk of developing type 2 diabetes mellitus. Journal of the American Medical Association. 2001;**286**(3):327-334

[65] Kopp HP et al. Impact of weight loss on inflammatory proteins and their association with the insulin resistance syndrome in morbidly obese patients. Arteriosclerosis, Thrombosis, and Vascular Biology. 2003;**23**(6):1042-1047

[66] Roytblat L et al. Raised interleukin-6 levels in obese patients. Obesity Research. 2000;**8**(9):673-675

[67] Laimer M et al. Markers of chronic inflammation and obesity: A prospective study on the reversibility of this association in middle-aged women undergoing weight loss by surgical intervention. International Journal of Obesity and Related Metabolic Disorders. 2002;**26**(5):659-662

[68] Bastard JP et al. Elevated levels of interleukin 6 are reduced in serum and subcutaneous adipose tissue of obese women after weight loss. The Journal of Clinical Endocrinology and Metabolism. 2000;**85**(9):3338-3342

[69] Yudkin JS et al. Inflammation, obesity, stress and coronary heart disease: Is interleukin-6 the link? Atherosclerosis. 2000;**148**(2):209-214

[70] Pepys MB, Hirschfield GM. C-reactive protein: A critical update. The Journal of Clinical Investigation. 2003;**111**(12):1805-1812

[71] Rotter V, Nagaev I, Smith U. Interleukin-6 (IL-6) induces insulin resistance in 3T3-L1 adipocytes and is, like IL-8 and tumor necrosis factor-alpha, overexpressed in human fat

cells from insulin-resistant subjects. The Journal of Biological Chemistry. 2003;**278**(46):45777-45784

[72] Fasshauer M et al. Adiponectin gene expression and secretion is inhibited by interleukin-6 in 3T3-L1 adipocytes. Biochemical and Biophysical Research Communications. 2003;**301**(4):1045-1050

[73] Senn JJ et al. Interleukin-6 induces cellular insulin resistance in hepatocytes. Diabetes. 2002;**51**(12):3391-3399

[74] Gustafson B, Smith U. Cytokines promote Wnt signaling and inflammation and impair the normal differentiation and lipid accumulation in 3T3-L1 preadipocytes. The Journal of Biological Chemistry. 2006;**281**(14):9507-9516

[75] Bing C. Is interleukin-1β a culprit in macrophage-adipocyte crosstalk in obesity? Adipocytes. 2015;**4**(2):149-152

[76] Labrecque J et al. Interleukin-1β and prostaglandin-synthesizing enzymes as modulators of human omental and subcutaneous adipose tissue function. Prostaglandins, Leukotrienes, and Essential Fatty Acids. 2019;**141**:9-16

[77] Bruun JM et al. Monocyte chemoattractant protein-1 release is higher in visceral than subcutaneous human adipose tissue (AT): Implication of macrophages resident in the AT. The Journal of Clinical Endocrinology and Metabolism. 2005;**90**(4):2282-2289

[78] Younce C, Kolattukudy P. MCP-1 induced protein promotes adipogenesis via oxidative stress, endoplasmic reticulum stress and autophagy. Cellular Physiology and Biochemistry : International Journal of Experimental Cellular Physiology, Biochemistry, and Pharmacology. 2012;**30**(2):307-320

[79] O'Rourke RW et al. Systemic inflammation and insulin sensitivity in obese IFN-γ knockout mice. Metabolism: Clinical and Experimental. 2012;**61**(8):1152-1161

[80] Harkins JM et al. Expression of interleukin-6 is greater in preadipocytes than in adipocytes of 3T3-L1 cells and C57BL/6J and Ob/Ob mice. The Journal of Nutrition. 2004;**134**(10):2673-2677

[81] Jung TW et al. β-Aminoisobutyric acid attenuates LPS-induced inflammation and insulin resistance in adipocytes through AMPK-mediated pathway. Journal of Biomedical Science. 2018;**25**(1):27

[82] Dang R-J et al. A20 plays a critical role in the immunoregulatory function of mesenchymal stem cells. Journal of Cellular and Molecular Medicine. 2016;**20**(8):1550-1560

[83] Ai L et al. A20 reduces lipid storage and inflammation in hypertrophic adipocytes via p38 and Akt signaling. Molecular and Cellular Biochemistry. 2016;**420**(1):73-83

[84] Liu Y et al. Nonerythropoietic erythropoietin-derived peptide suppresses adipogenesis, inflammation, obesity and insulin resistance. Scientific Reports. 2015;**5**:15134

[85] Ahlqvist E et al. Link between GIP and osteopontin in adipose tissue and insulin resistance. Diabetes. 2013;**62**(6):2088-2094

[86] Li X et al. Bio-informatics analysis of a gene co-expression module in adipose tissue containing the diet-responsive gene Nnat. BMC Systems Biology. 2010;**4**:175

[87] Higuchi M et al. Differentiation of human adipose-derived stem cells into fat involves reactive oxygen species and Forkhead box O1 mediated upregulation of antioxidant enzymes. Stem Cells and Development. 2013;**22**(6):878-888

[88] Liu R et al. Dynamic differences in oxidative stress and the regulation of metabolism with age in visceral versus subcutaneous adipose. Redox Biology. 2015;**6**:401-408

[89] Okuno Y et al. Oxidative stress inhibits healthy adipose expansion through suppression of SREBF1-mediated lipogenic pathway. Diabetes. 2018;**67**(6):1113-1127

[90] Tchkonia T et al. Fat tissue, aging, and cellular senescence. Aging Cell. 2010;**9**(5):667-684

[91] Furukawa S et al. Increased oxidative stress in obesity and its impact on metabolic syndrome. The Journal of Clinical Investigation. 2004;**114**(12):1752-1761

[92] Gueraud F et al. Chemistry and biochemistry of lipid peroxidation products. Free Radical Research. 2010;**44**(10):1098-1124

[93] Salans LB, Knittle JL, Hirsch J. The role of adipose cell size and adipose tissue insulin sensitivity in the carbohydrate intolerance of human obesity. The Journal of Clinical Investigation. 1968;**47**(1):153-165

[94] Higdon A et al. Cell signalling by reactive lipid species: New concepts and molecular mechanisms. The Biochemical Journal. 2012;**442**(3):453-464

[95] Bauer G, Zarkovic N. Revealing mechanisms of selective, concentration-dependent potentials of 4-hydroxy-2-nonenal to induce apoptosis in cancer cells through inactivation of membrane-associated catalase. Free Radical Biology and Medicine. 2015;**81**:128-144

[96] Chen ZH, Niki E. 4-hydroxynonenal (4-HNE) has been widely accepted as an inducer of oxidative stress. Is this the whole truth about it or can 4-HNE also exert protective effects? IUBMB Life. 2006;**58**(5-6):372-373

[97] Huh JY et al. 8-Hydroxy-2-deoxyguanosine ameliorates high-fat diet-induced insulin resistance and adipocyte dysfunction in mice. Biochemical and Biophysical Research Communications. 2017;**491**(4):890-896

[98] Murdolo G et al. Free radical-derived oxysterols: Novel adipokines modulating adipogenic differentiation of adipose precursor cells. The Journal of Clinical Endocrinology and Metabolism. 2016;**101**(12):4974-4983

[99] Vanella L et al. Increased heme-oxygenase 1 expression in mesenchymal stem cell-derived adipocytes decreases differentiation and lipid accumulation via upregulation of the canonical Wnt signaling cascade. Stem Cell Research and Therapy. 2013;**4**(2):28

[100] Lin C-H et al. Oxidative stress induces imbalance of adipogenic/osteoblastic lineage commitment in mesenchymal stem cells through decreasing SIRT1 functions. Journal of Cellular and Molecular Medicine. 2018;**22**(2):786-796

[101] Denu RA, Hematti P. Effects of oxidative stress on mesenchymal stem cell biology. Oxidative Medicine and Cellular Longevity. 2016;**2016**:2989076

[102] Puri N et al. Heme induced oxidative stress attenuates sirtuin1 and enhances adipogenesis in mesenchymal stem cells and mouse pre-adipocytes. Journal of Cellular Biochemistry. 2012;**113**(6):1926-1935

[103] Moreno-Navarrete JM et al. Deleted in breast cancer 1 plays a functional role in adipocyte differentiation. American Journal of Physiology. Endocrinology and Metabolism. 2015;**308**(7):E554-E561

[104] Wu Y-T et al. Depletion of Sirt3 leads to the impairment of adipogenic differentiation and insulin resistance via interfering mitochondrial function of

adipose-derived human mesenchymal stem cells. Free Radical Research. 2018;**52**(11):1398-1415

[105] Chang Y-C et al. Deficiency of NPGPx, an oxidative stress sensor, leads to obesity in mice and human. EMBO Molecular Medicine. 2013;**5**(8):1165-1179

[106] Castro JP, Grune T, Speckmann B. The two faces of reactive oxygen species (ROS) in adipocyte function and dysfunction. Biological Chemistry. 2016;**397**(8):709-724

[107] Alcala M et al. Short-term vitamin E treatment impairs reactive oxygen species signaling required for adipose tissue expansion, resulting in fatty liver and insulin resistance in obese mice. PLoS One. 2017;**12**(10):e0186579

[108] Pieralisi A et al. N-acetylcysteine inhibits lipid accumulation in mouse embryonic adipocytes. Redox Biology. 2016;**9**:39-44

[109] Peris E et al. Antioxidant treatment induces reductive stress associated with mitochondrial dysfunction in adipocytes. The Journal of Biological Chemistry. 2019;**294**(7):2340-2352

[110] Findeisen HM et al. Oxidative stress accumulates in adipose tissue during aging and inhibits adipogenesis. PLoS One. 2011;**6**(4):e18532

[111] Zhang C, Klett EL, Coleman RA. Lipid signals and insulin resistance. Journal of Clinical Lipidology. 2013;**8**(6):659-667

[112] Jiao P et al. FFA-induced adipocyte inflammation and insulin resistance: Involvement of ER stress and IKKbeta pathways. Obesity (Silver Spring). 2011;**19**(3):483-491

[113] Furuhashi M, Hotamisligil GS. Fatty acid-binding proteins: Role in metabolic diseases and potential as drug targets. Nature Reviews. Drug Discovery. 2008;**7**(6):489-503

[114] Summers SA. Ceramides in insulin resistance and lipotoxicity. Progress in Lipid Research. 2006;**45**(1):42-72

[115] Barbarroja N et al. Increased dihydroceramide/ceramide ratio mediated by defective expression of degs1 impairs adipocyte differentiation and function. Diabetes. 2015;**64**(4):1180-1192

[116] Papackova Z, Cahova M. Fatty acid signaling: The new function of intracellular lipases. International Journal of Molecular Sciences. 2015;**16**(2):3831-3855

[117] Roy D et al. Coordinated transcriptional control of adipocyte triglyceride lipase (Atgl) by transcription factors Sp1 and peroxisome proliferator-activated receptor γ (PPARγ) during adipocyte differentiation. The Journal of Biological Chemistry. 2017;**292**(36):14827-14835

[118] Clarke SD. Polyunsaturated fatty acid regulation of gene transcription: A molecular mechanism to improve the metabolic syndrome. The Journal of Nutrition. 2001;**131**(4):1129-1132

[119] Clarke SD. The multi-dimensional regulation of gene expression by fatty acids: Polyunsaturated fats as nutrient sensors. Current Opinion in Lipidology. 2004;**15**(1):13-18

[120] Kersten S. Effects of fatty acids on gene expression: Role of peroxisome proliferator-activated receptor alpha, liver X receptor alpha and sterol regulatory element-binding protein-1c. The Proceedings of the Nutrition Society. 2002;**61**(3):371-374

[121] Wahle KW, Rotondo D, Heys SD. Polyunsaturated fatty acids and gene expression in mammalian systems. The Proceedings of the Nutrition Society. 2003;**62**(2):349-360

[122] Forman BM, Chen J, Evans RM. Hypolipidemic drugs, polyunsaturated fatty acids, and eicosanoids are ligands for peroxisome proliferator-activated receptors alpha and delta. Proceedings of the National Academy of Sciences of the United States of America. 1997;**94**(9):4312-4317

[123] Johnson TE et al. Structural requirements and cell-type specificity for ligand activation of peroxisome proliferator-activated receptors. The Journal of Steroid Biochemistry and Molecular Biology. 1997;**63**(1):1-8

[124] Yu K et al. Differential activation of peroxisome proliferator-activated receptors by eicosanoids. Journal of Biological Chemistry. 1995;**270**(41):23975-23983

[125] Kliewer SA et al. Fatty acids and eicosanoids regulate gene expression through direct interactions with peroxisome proliferator-activated receptors alpha and gamma. Proceedings of the National Academy of Sciences of the United States of America. 1997;**94**(9):4318-4323

[126] Keller H et al. Fatty acids and retinoids control lipid metabolism through activation of peroxisome proliferator-activated receptor-retinoid X receptor heterodimers. Proceedings of the National Academy of Sciences of the United States of America. 1993;**90**(6):2160-2164

[127] Roynette CE et al. n-3 polyunsaturated fatty acids and colon cancer prevention. Clinical Nutrition. 2004;**23**(2):139-151

[128] Hirafuji M et al. Cardiovascular protective effects of n-3 polyunsaturated fatty acids with special emphasis on docosahexaenoic acid. Journal of Pharmacological Sciences. 2003;**92**(4):308-316

[129] Abeywardena MY, Head RJ. Long-chain n-3 polyunsaturated fatty acids and blood vessel function. Cardiovascular Research. 2001;**52**(3):361-371

[130] Bucher HC et al. N-3 polyunsaturated fatty acids in coronary heart disease: A meta-analysis of randomized controlled trials. The American Journal of Medicine. 2002;**112**(4):298-304

[131] Larsson SC et al. Dietary long-chain n-3 fatty acids for the prevention of cancer: A review of potential mechanisms. The American Journal of Clinical Nutrition. 2004;**79**(6):935-945

[132] Worgall TS et al. Polyunsaturated fatty acids decrease expression of promoters with sterol regulatory elements by decreasing levels of mature sterol regulatory element-binding protein. The Journal of Biological Chemistry. 1998;**273**(40):25537-25540

[133] Hannah VC et al. Unsaturated fatty acids down-regulate srebp isoforms 1a and 1c by two mechanisms in HEK-293 cells. Journal of Biological Chemistry. 2001;**276**(6):4365-4372

[134] Mater MK et al. Sterol response element-binding protein 1c (SREBP1c) is involved in the polyunsaturated fatty acid suppression of hepatic S14 gene transcription. Journal of Biological Chemistry. 1999;**274**(46):32725-32732

[135] Xu J et al. Sterol regulatory element binding protein-1 expression is suppressed by dietary polyunsaturated fatty acids. A mechanism for the coordinate suppression of lipogenic genes by polyunsaturated fats. Journal of Biological Chemistry. 1999;**274**(33):23577-23583

[136] Ou J et al. Unsaturated fatty acids inhibit transcription of the sterol regulatory element-binding protein-1c (SREBP-1c) gene by antagonizing ligand-dependent activation of the LXR. Proceedings

of the National Academy of Sciences. 2001;**98**(11):6027-6032

[137] Yoshikawa T et al. Polyunsaturated fatty acids suppress sterol regulatory element-binding protein 1c promoter activity by inhibition of liver X receptor (LXR) binding to LXR response elements. The Journal of Biological Chemistry. 2002;**277**(3):1705-1711

[138] Barak Y et al. PPAR gamma is required for placental, cardiac, and adipose tissue development. Molecular Cell. 1999;**4**(4):585-595

[139] Göttlicher M et al. Structural and metabolic requirements for activators of the peroxisome proliferator-activated receptor. Biochemical Pharmacology. 1993;**46**(12):2177-2184

[140] Nakamura MT et al. Mechanisms of regulation of gene expression by fatty acids. Lipids. 2004;**39**(11):1077-1083

[141] Cho K-J et al. Alpha-lipoic acid inhibits adipocyte differentiation by regulating pro-adipogenic transcription factors via mitogen-activated protein kinase pathways. The Journal of Biological Chemistry. 2003;**278**(37):34823-34833

[142] Goto T et al. 10-oxo-12(Z)-octadecenoic acid, a linoleic acid metabolite produced by gut lactic acid bacteria, potently activates PPARγ and stimulates adipogenesis. Biochemical and Biophysical Research Communications. 2015;**459**(4):597-603

[143] Wong SH et al. The adaptive effects of dietary fish and safflower oil on lipid and lipoprotein metabolism in perfused rat liver. Biochimica et Biophysica Acta. 1984;**792**(2):103-109

[144] Ren B et al. Polyunsaturated fatty acid suppression of hepatic fatty acid synthase and S14 gene expression does not require peroxisome proliferator-activated receptor alpha. The Journal of Biological Chemistry. 1997;**272**(43):26827-26832

[145] Rustan AC, Christiansen EN, Drevon CA. Serum lipids, hepatic glycerolipid metabolism and peroxisomal fatty acid oxidation in rats fed omega-3 and omega-6 fatty acids. The Biochemical Journal. 1992;**283**(Pt 2):333-339

[146] Takeuchi H et al. Comparative effects of dietary fat types on hepatic enzyme activities related to the synthesis and oxidation of fatty acid and to lipogenesis in rats. Bioscience, Biotechnology, and Biochemistry. 2001;**65**(8):1748-1754

[147] Madsen L, Petersen RK, Kristiansen K. Regulation of adipocyte differentiation and function by polyunsaturated fatty acids. Biochimica et Biophysica Acta. 2005;**1740**(2):266-286

[148] Jove M et al. Human omental and subcutaneous adipose tissue exhibit specific lipidomic signatures. The FASEB Journal. 2014;**28**(3):1071-1081

[149] Hodson L, Skeaff CM, Fielding BA. Fatty acid composition of adipose tissue and blood in humans and its use as a biomarker of dietary intake. Progress in Lipid Research. 2008;**47**(5):348-380

[150] Denys A, Hichami A, Khan NA. Eicosapentaenoic acid and docosahexaenoic acid modulate MAP kinase enzyme activity in human T-cells. Molecular and Cellular Biochemistry. 2002;**232**(1-2):143-148

[151] Fan X et al. Arachidonic acid and related methyl ester mediate protein kinase C activation in intact platelets through the arachidonate metabolism pathways. Biochemical and Biophysical Research Communications. 1990;**169**(3):933-940

[152] Jiang YH et al. Dietary fat and fiber differentially alter intracellular second

messengers during tumor development in rat colon. Carcinogenesis. 1996;**17**(6):1227-1233

[153] Kawaguchi T et al. Mechanism for fatty acid "sparing" effect on glucose-induced transcription: Regulation of carbohydrate-responsive element-binding protein by AMP-activated protein kinase. The Journal of Biological Chemistry. 2002;**277**(6):3829-3835

[154] Murata M et al. Dual action of eicosapentaenoic acid in hepatoma cells: Up-regulation of metabolic action of insulin and inhibition of cell proliferation. The Journal of Biological Chemistry. 2001;**276**(33):31422-31428

[155] Madani S et al. Diacylglycerols containing omega 3 and omega 6 fatty acids bind to RasGRP and modulate MAP kinase activation. The Journal of Biological Chemistry. 2004;**279**(2):1176-1183

[156] Nikolopoulou E et al. Arachidonic acid-dependent gene regulation during preadipocyte differentiation controls adipocyte potential. Journal of Lipid Research. 2014;**55**(12):2479-2490

[157] Moreno-Santos I et al. The antagonist effect of arachidonic acid on GLUT4 gene expression by nuclear receptor type II regulation. International Journal of Molecular Sciences. 2019;**20**(4):963

[158] Catalioto RM et al. Autocrine control of adipose cell differentiation by prostacyclin and PGF2 alpha. Biochimica et Biophysica Acta. 1991;**1091**(3):364-369

[159] Gaillard D et al. Requirement and role of arachidonic acid in the differentiation of pre-adipose cells. The Biochemical Journal. 1989;**257**(2):389-397

[160] Negrel R, Gaillard D, Ailhaud G. Prostacyclin as a potent effector of adipose-cell differentiation. The Biochemical Journal. 1989;**257**(2):399-405

[161] Forman BM et al. 15-Deoxy-delta 12, 14-prostaglandin J2 is a ligand for the adipocyte determination factor PPAR gamma. Cell. 1995;**83**(5):803-812

[162] Kliewer SA et al. A prostaglandin J2 metabolite binds peroxisome proliferator-activated receptor gamma and promotes adipocyte differentiation. Cell. 1995;**83**(5):813-819

[163] Serrero G, Lepak NM. Prostaglandin F2alpha receptor (FP receptor) agonists are potent adipose differentiation inhibitors for primary culture of adipocyte precursors in defined medium. Biochemical and Biophysical Research Communications. 1997;**233**(1):200-202

[164] Serrero G, Lepak NM, Goodrich SP. Paracrine regulation of adipose differentiation by arachidonate metabolites: Prostaglandin F2 alpha inhibits early and late markers of differentiation in the adipogenic cell line 1246. Endocrinology. 1992;**131**(6):2545-2551

[165] Serrero G, Lepak NM, Goodrich SP. Prostaglandin F2 alpha inhibits the differentiation of adipocyte precursors in primary culture. Biochemical and Biophysical Research Communications. 1992;**183**(2):438-442

[166] Casimir DA, Miller CW, Ntambi JM. Preadipocyte differentiation blocked by prostaglandin stimulation of prostanoid FP2 receptor in murine 3T3-L1 cells. Differentiation. 1996;**60**(4):203-210

[167] Kamon J et al. Prostaglandin F(2)alpha enhances glucose consumption through neither adipocyte differentiation nor GLUT1 expression in 3T3-L1 cells. Cellular Signalling. 2001;**13**(2):105-109

[168] Miller CW, Casimir DA, Ntambi JM. The mechanism of inhibition of 3T3-L1 preadipocyte differentiation by prostaglandin F2alpha. Endocrinology. 1996;**137**(12):5641-5650

[169] Reginato MJ et al. Prostaglandins promote and block adipogenesis through opposing effects on peroxisome proliferator-activated receptor gamma. The Journal of Biological Chemistry. 1998;**273**(4):1855-1858

[170] Vassaux G et al. Differential response of preadipocytes and adipocytes to prostacyclin and prostaglandin E2: Physiological implications. Endocrinology. 1992;**131**(5):2393-2398

[171] Sugimoto Y et al. Microarray evaluation of EP4 receptor-mediated prostaglandin E2 suppression of 3T3-L1 adipocyte differentiation. Biochemical and Biophysical Research Communications. 2004;**322**(3):911-917

[172] Tsuboi H et al. Prostanoid EP4 receptor is involved in suppression of 3T3-L1 adipocyte differentiation. Biochemical and Biophysical Research Communications. 2004;**322**(3):1066-1072

[173] Li R et al. CYP2J2 attenuates metabolic dysfunction in diabetic mice by reducing hepatic inflammation via the PPARγ. American Journal of Physiology. Endocrinology and Metabolism. 2015;**308**(4):E270-E282

[174] Suzuki M, Tamura T, Shimomura Y. Less body fat accumulation in rats fed a safflower oil diet than in rats fed a beef tallow diet. The Journal of Nutrition. 1990;**120**(11):1291-1296

[175] Wang H, Storlien LH, Huang X-F. Effects of dietary fat types on body fatness, leptin, and ARC leptin receptor, NPY, and AgRP mRNA expression. American Journal of Physiology-Endocrinology and Metabolism. 2002;**282**(6):E1352-E1359

[176] Minami A et al. Effect of eicosapentaenoic acid ethyl ester v. oleic acid-rich safflower oil on insulin resistance in type 2 diabetic model rats with hypertriacylglycerolaemia. The British Journal of Nutrition. 2002;**87**(2):157-162

[177] Cha SH et al. Chronic docosahexaenoic acid intake enhances expression of the gene for uncoupling protein 3 and affects pleiotropic mRNA levels in skeletal muscle of aged C57BL/6NJcl mice. The Journal of Nutrition. 2001;**131**(10):2636-2642

[178] Takahashi Y, Ide T. Dietary n-3 fatty acids affect mRNA level of brown adipose tissue uncoupling protein 1, and white adipose tissue leptin and glucose transporter 4 in the rat. The British Journal of Nutrition. 2000;**84**(2):175-184

[179] Okuno M et al. Perilla oil prevents the excessive growth of visceral adipose tissue in rats by down-regulating adipocyte differentiation. The Journal of Nutrition. 1997;**127**(9):1752-1757

[180] Jang IS et al. Role of dietary fat type in the development of adiposity from dietary obesity-susceptible Sprague-Dawley rats. The British Journal of Nutrition. 2003;**89**(3):429-438

[181] Nakatani T et al. A low fish oil inhibits SREBP-1 proteolytic cascade, while a high-fish-oil feeding decreases SREBP-1 mRNA in mice liver: Relationship to anti-obesity. Journal of Lipid Research. 2003;**44**(2):369-379

[182] Ukropec J et al. The hypotriglyceridemic effect of dietary n-3 FA is associated with increased beta-oxidation and reduced leptin expression. Lipids. 2003;**38**(10):1023-1029

[183] Pellizzon M et al. Effects of dietary fatty acids and exercise on body-weight regulation and metabolism in rats. Obesity Research. 2002;**10**(9):947-955

[184] Liberato MV et al. Medium chain fatty acids are selective peroxisome proliferator activated receptor (PPAR) γ activators and pan-PPAR partial agonists. PLoS One. 2012;7(5):e36297

[185] Senarath S et al. Comparison of the effects of long-chain monounsaturated fatty acid positional isomers on lipid metabolism in 3T3-L1 cells. Journal of Oleo Science. 2019

[186] Zhao G et al. Anti-inflammatory effects of polyunsaturated fatty acids in THP-1 cells. Biochemical and Biophysical Research Communications. 2005;**336**(3):909-917

[187] Amri EZ, Ailhaud G, Grimaldi PA. Fatty acids as signal transducing molecules: Involvement in the differentiation of preadipose to adipose cells. Journal of Lipid Research. 1994;**35**(5):930-937

[188] Davies JD et al. Adipocytic differentiation and liver x receptor pathways regulate the accumulation of triacylglycerols in human vascular smooth muscle cells. The Journal of Biological Chemistry. 2005;**280**(5):3911-3919

[189] Ding S, Mersmann HJ. Fatty acids modulate porcine adipocyte differentiation and transcripts for transcription factors and adipocyte-characteristic proteins*. The Journal of Nutritional Biochemistry. 2001;**12**(2):101-108

[190] McNeel RL, Mersmann HJ. Effects of isomers of conjugated linoleic acid on porcine adipocyte growth and differentiation. The Journal of Nutritional Biochemistry. 2003;**14**(5):266-274

[191] Wolins NE et al. S3-12, Adipophilin, and TIP47 package lipid in adipocytes. The Journal of Biological Chemistry. 2005;**280**(19):19146-19155

[192] Magliano DJ et al. Persistent organic pollutants and diabetes: A review of the epidemiological evidence. Diabetes and Metabolism. 2014;**40**(1):1-14

[193] Farkhondeh T, Samarghandian S, Azimi-Nezhad M. The role of arsenic in obesity and diabetes. Journal of Cellular Physiology. 2019 Aug;**234**(8):12516-12529

[194] Bartlett DE et al. Uremic toxins activates Na/K-ATPase oxidant amplification loop causing phenotypic changes in adipocytes in In vitro models. International Journal of Molecular Sciences. 2018;**19**(9):2685

[195] Milton FA et al. Dibutyltin compounds effects on PPARγ/RXRα activity, adipogenesis, and inflammation in mammalians cells. Frontiers in Pharmacology. 2017;**8**:507